Gastroenterology

Nursing Care

The Complete Guide

ALEXANDRE CAREWELL

Table of Contents

« *The journey through the digestive system is an exploration into the heart of our being; in gastroenterology, we discover that health begins from within.* »

Chapter 1
INTRODUCTION
GASTROENTEROLOGY

Definition and general presentation of the speciality.

Gastroenterology, a word as complex sounding as the speciality itself, is the branch of medicine devoted to the study, diagnosis, treatment and prevention of diseases affecting the digestive system. It covers everything to do with the oesophagus, stomach, small intestine, colon, rectum, pancreas, liver and gallbladder. But what makes it so special, so distinct from other medical disciplines?

Imagine a marvellously designed system, a series of interconnected organs and ducts that transform the food we eat into the nutrients essential to our survival, while evacuating what is superfluous. That's the magic of our digestive system. Gastroenterology is the window that opens onto this fascinating internal world, enabling health professionals to understand its mysteries, treat its ailments and optimise its functioning.

But gastroenterology doesn't stop there. It also reflects our lifestyles, eating habits and many other environmental factors that can influence our digestive well-being. The richness of this speciality lies in its ability to blend pure science with a holistic approach to health, always seeking to understand the patient as a whole.
Far from being confined to the confines of hospitals, gastroenterology also extends to clinics, doctors' surgeries and even research centres. It is constantly evolving, driven by technological and scientific advances that are

constantly pushing back the boundaries of what we know and what we can do for the well-being of our patients.

In short, gastroenterology is much more than just a medical speciality. It is a witness to the history of each individual, a subtle dance between anatomy, physiology, psychology and the environment in which we live. And that's what makes it such an exciting and essential part of the vast medical panorama.

Historical overview: developments in the field.

Tracing the history of gastroenterology back in time is a bit like following the winding course of a river, rich in twists and turns, discoveries and innovations. Long before the very term 'gastroenterology' was coined, ancient civilisations were already pondering the mysteries of the digestive system. From Egyptian papyri to Indian Ayurvedic treatises, via the texts of Hippocrates in ancient Greece, interest in digestive well-being and the diseases associated with it is ancestral.

However, it was only in the 19th century, with the advent of modern medicine, that gastroenterology really took off as a specialist discipline. The invention of the gastroscope, an instrument that for the first time allowed direct visualization of the interior of the stomach, marked a decisive turning point. Instead of relying on guesswork, doctors were now able to make precise diagnoses and propose more appropriate treatments.

The 20th century saw a flurry of innovations. Endoscopy, for example, has seen major advances, making it possible to explore not only the oesophagus and stomach, but also the colon, radically transforming the way in which many conditions are diagnosed and treated. Similarly, advances in molecular biology and genetics have offered invaluable insights into chronic inflammatory bowel diseases such as Crohn's disease and haemorrhagic rectocolitis.

But while technology and research have largely contributed to shaping gastroenterology, the role of patients themselves should not be underestimated. Their desire to be better informed, their desire for more personalised care, have also influenced developments in the field. Patient movements, such as those fighting hepatitis, have given a voice to those who previously felt marginalised or misunderstood.

Today, gastroenterology is at a crossroads. With the explosion of data and the digital revolution, the era of personalised medicine is on the horizon. Understanding microbiomes, the complex ecosystems of micro-organisms living in our digestive system, promises to revolutionise once again our approach to gastrointestinal diseases.

Revisiting the history of gastroenterology means embracing a rich, complex and promising heritage. It means understanding that behind every discovery, every advance, there is an unshakeable desire to improve the lives of patients and to unlock the secrets of a system that is as fascinating as it is essential to our existence.

The importance of gastroenterology in the medical field.

Gastroenterology, although it may seem specialised, occupies a central place in the vast medical universe. This speciality reflects the complexity and fundamental importance of the digestive system to our general well-being. To understand its crucial importance, we need only consider a number of dimensions.

Firstly, from a purely physiological point of view, the digestive system is responsible for the transformation and assimilation of nutrients, processes which are essential to our survival. But beyond this vital function, the intestine, often called 'the second brain', is a major hub of neurotransmitters and is intimately linked to our nervous system. It is with this in mind that gastroenterology also interacts with neurology, particularly in understanding the links between intestinal health and conditions such as depression or anxiety.

Secondly, the liver, one of the major organs studied in gastroenterology, plays a pivotal role in detoxifying the body, producing bile and regulating metabolism. Liver diseases, such as hepatitis or cirrhosis, can have systemic consequences, impacting other organs and requiring a multidisciplinary approach.

In addition, gastroenterology is at the heart of some of the world's most prevalent and growing diseases, such as chronic inflammatory bowel disease, gastro-oesophageal reflux disease and cancers of the digestive system. Treating these conditions requires cutting-edge expertise, advanced technologies and close collaboration with other specialists such as surgeons, radiologists or oncologists.

But it's not just the disease. Gastroenterology also plays a major preventive role. Colorectal cancer screening campaigns, for example, have saved countless lives by detecting and treating precancerous lesions.

Finally, gastroenterology is also a gateway to understanding the intestinal microbiota, the vast array of micro-organisms living in symbiosis with us. Recent research shows that this microbiota influences not only our digestive health, but also our immunity, our metabolism and even our behaviour.

In short, gastroenterology is not just another medical speciality. It is a crossroads, an intersection between various disciplines, testifying to the profound interdependence of our bodily systems. It embodies the very essence of medicine: a never-ending quest to understand the whole human being, always seeking to improve the quality of life.

Chapter 2
THE WORKING ENVIRONMENT:
A SERVICE LIKE NO OTHER

Presentation of
the gastroenterology unit.

At the heart of every hospital dedicated to specialist care is the gastroenterology unit, a haven dedicated to the exploration, diagnosis and treatment of diseases linked to the digestive system. This unit, which is both a state-of-the-art laboratory and a sanctuary of care, is the hub around which the entire speciality revolves. Here's a look at this complex and fascinating world.

The gastroenterology unit is distinguished first and foremost by its adapted infrastructure. Often equipped with the latest technology, it includes endoscopy rooms where doctors can perform invasive explorations such as colonoscopy, gastroscopy or biliary endoscopy. Each room is designed to ensure patient safety and comfort, while enabling the practitioner to work with precision.

There is also an inpatient wing. Here, patients suffering from more serious illnesses or requiring constant monitoring can be cared for. Whether it's for acute pancreatitis, a severe flare-up of inflammatory bowel disease or after digestive surgery, this wing is essential to ensure comprehensive patient care.

But the gastroenterology unit is more than just walls and machines. Above all, it's a team. Expert gastroenterologists, of course, but also specialist nurses, trained to understand the specificities of digestive diseases and to administer appropriate care. There are also Caregivers, technicians, medical secretaries and many other professionals who contribute to the smooth running of the unit.

In addition, the gastroenterology unit often has close links with other departments. Collaboration with the digestive surgery department is frequent, as is interaction with radiologists for imaging examinations or with oncologists for the management of digestive cancers.

An aspect that is sometimes overlooked, but just as crucial, is research. Many gastroenterology units are involved in clinical trials, seeking to develop new treatments or better understand the underlying mechanisms of disease.
In addition to its technical expertise, the gastroenterology unit is also a place of humanity. Every patient is given a warm welcome, and every story is listened to carefully. Because while medicine is a science, it is above all an art, the art of caring with the heart.

So the gastroenterology unit, far from being just another department, reflects the complexity and richness of the speciality itself. A place where science, technology, care and humanity come together to offer the best to those who need it most.

Specific equipment and their use.

One of the fascinating aspects of gastroenterology is the variety and sophistication of the equipment used. These instruments, the fruit of years of research and innovation, enable specialists to diagnose, treat and monitor gastrointestinal disorders with precision. Here is a presentation of the main equipment and how it is used.

- **Endoscope**: This is a long flexible tube fitted with a camera and a light source at the end. It is inserted through the patient's mouth or anus.
  - **Gastroscopy**: Use of an endoscope to examine the oesophagus, stomach and beginning of the duodenum.
  - **Colonoscopy**: examination of the colon and possibly the rectum.
  - **Enteroscopy**: Examination of the deeper parts of the small intestine.
- **Echoendoscope**: A combination of an endoscope and an ultrasound scanner. It is used to obtain ultrasound images of internal structures close to the digestive tract, such as the pancreas or bile.
  - **Echoendoscopy**: Used to assess tumours, cysts or other abnormalities and can also be used to take tissue samples.
- **Endoscopic capsule**: A small capsule containing a camera, swallowed by the patient. It passes through the digestive system, sending wireless images for evaluation.
  - Mainly used to visualise the small intestine, an area that is difficult to reach with conventional endoscopes.
- **Manometer**: device used to measure the pressure inside certain segments of the digestive tract.
  - **Oesophageal manometry**: assesses the motility of the oesophagus, useful for conditions such as achalasia.
- **PH-meter:** A device that measures the level of acidity (pH) in the oesophagus over a prolonged period.
  - Used to diagnose gastro-oesophageal reflux disease.
- **Double balloon endoscope**: An advanced endoscopic system that uses two balloons to anchor

the device and progressively advance into the small intestine.

- Allows exploration of the entire small intestine.
- **Radiofrequency Ablation (RFA) System**: Used to treat precancerous lesions in the oesophagus, such as dysplasia in Barrett's oesophagus.
- **Elastic ligation equipment**: Used to treat oesophageal varices by ligating bleeding vessels.

Each piece of equipment requires specific training and expertise if it is to be used correctly and safely. Beyond the technology, choosing the right equipment and mastering its use are essential to making an accurate diagnosis and proposing appropriate treatment. Gastroenterology, with its sophisticated instruments, is a perfect example of how modern technology can be used to improve patient care.

Multidisciplinarity : collaboration with other departments.

Gastroenterology, with its richness and complexity, cannot be isolated from other medical disciplines. Each patient, each disease, may require expertise that goes beyond the strict boundaries of the specialty. Multidisciplinarity is not only desirable, it is essential if patients are to be treated holistically and optimally. Here's a closer look at this crucial collaboration with other departments.

- **Digestive surgery**: This collaboration is one of the most obvious. Whether for gastrointestinal tumours, obstructions or complications of inflammatory bowel disease, the digestive surgeon works hand in hand with the gastroenterologist to offer the best therapeutic strategy.

- **Radiology**: Imaging plays a central role in the diagnosis of gastrointestinal diseases. Whether it's an abdominal ultrasound, an enteric MRI or a CT scan, the radiologist is often the first to detect an abnormality, which is then treated by the gastroenterologist.
- **Oncology**: Cancers of the digestive system require collaborative management. The oncologist proposes chemotherapy or immunotherapy strategies, while the gastroenterologist monitors the progress of the disease and manages complications.
- **Pathology**: Using microscope slides, the pathologist confirms or refutes a diagnosis of cancer, inflammatory disease or other digestive pathologies. Collaboration is crucial, particularly during multidisciplinary consultation meetings.
- **Rheumatology**: Certain disorders, such as ankylosing spondylitis, can be associated with inflammatory bowel disease. Coordination between the rheumatologist and the gastroenterologist is essential for comprehensive care.
- **Dermatology**: Conditions such as psoriasis can be linked to gastrointestinal disorders, requiring a joint approach.
- **Endocrinology**: Liver diseases such as steatosis are closely linked to metabolic disorders, which is why it is so important to work with an endocrinologist.
- **Psychiatry and psychology**: Mental health and digestive health are more closely linked than is often realised. Irritable bowel syndrome, for example, can be exacerbated by stress or anxiety. Collaboration with mental health specialists is sometimes essential for comprehensive management.
- **Nutrition**: Dietetics and nutrition are at the heart of gastroenterology. Whether to manage malabsorption or intolerance, or to advise on a specific diet, the nutritionist or dietician is a valuable ally.

This multidisciplinary approach reflects the complexity of the human condition. Each speciality and each department makes its own contribution, ensuring that every patient benefits from a 360° view of their illness and the best therapeutic strategies. In this complex and harmonious dance, the gastroenterologist, while a specialist, is also a coordinator, a conductor at the heart of medicine.

Chapter 3
THE CENTRAL ROLE OF THE NURSE IN GASTROENTEROLOGY

The specificities of the nursing role in this department.

The role of the gastroenterology nurse is complex, demanding and rewarding. At the heart of care, the nurse is often the first and last point of contact for patients, offering both technical care and emotional support. Let's explore the specifics of this essential role.

- **Specific technical care**: Gastroenterology nurses must master a range of technical skills specific to the speciality.
  - **Preparing for the endoscopy**: This includes administering lavage solutions, taking a medical history and checking current medication.
  - **Assistance during endoscopic procedures**: Working with the gastroenterologist to ensure that the examination runs smoothly and safely.
  - **Post-procedural management**: Monitoring vital signs, managing potential complications and offering advice on post-procedural care.
- **Patient education**: Nurses play an essential educational role, helping patients to understand their condition, their treatments and how they can manage their health at home.
  - Advice on diet, medication and preventing complications.

- **Emotional support**: Gastrointestinal disorders can have a profound impact on patients' quality of life. The nurse offers psychological support, listening to patients' concerns and reassuring them.
- **Care coordination**: The nurse acts as a pivot between the patient, the specialist doctor and other health professionals, ensuring fluid communication and holistic care.
- **Clinical research**: In some units, nurses may be involved in research, helping to set up clinical studies, collect data or monitor participating patients.
- **Management of special therapies**: This may include administering biological treatments for conditions such as Crohn's disease or ulcerative colitis, or managing patients on enteral or parenteral nutrition.
- **Infection prevention**: Due to the invasive nature of many gastroenterology procedures, nurses play a crucial role in infection prevention, ensuring that equipment is sterilised and hygiene protocols are strictly followed.
- **Continuing education**: The field of gastroenterology is evolving rapidly. Nurses must therefore engage in ongoing training to keep abreast of the latest advances and best practices.

In the final analysis, the gastroenterology nurse is much more than a simple operator. They are the guardians of patient safety, the educators, the confidants and often the intermediaries between the medical world and the patient. In this specialty, as in many others, the nurse is the beating heart of the department, ensuring that every patient is treated with competence, compassion and dignity.

The skills and qualities required.

Gastroenterology nurses, as in other medical specialities, need a combination of technical, interpersonal and intellectual skills to excel in their role. Here are the essential skills and qualities for a nurse in this field:

- Solid clinical skills:
    - Mastery of drug administration techniques, post-operative care and procedures specific to gastroenterology.
    - Ability to carry out detailed clinical assessments and interpret data to guide management.
- Communication skills :
    - Ability to explain complex conditions and procedures in a way that patients can understand.
    - Active listening to understand patients' concerns and needs.
- Empathy and compassion:
    - Sensitivity to patients' personal and emotional problems, particularly when faced with difficult diagnoses or invasive treatments.
- Stress management :
    - Ability to remain calm and organised in stressful or emergency situations.

- Teamwork :
    - Ability to work in collaboration with gastroenterologists, surgeons, Caregivers, nutritionists and other healthcare professionals.
- Problem-solving and decision-making :
    - Ability to assess a situation quickly, consider different solutions and make informed decisions.

- Updating knowledge :
    - Commitment to continuing education and keeping abreast of the latest research and innovations in gastroenterology.
- Manual dexterity :
    - For precise   handling of specific medical instruments or equipment.
- Confidentiality :
    - Strict respect for patients' rights to confidentiality and data protection.
- Organisation and time management :
- Ability to prioritise tasks effectively in a fast-paced environment and to manage several requests simultaneously.
- Strong professional ethics :
- Commitment to professional standards, integrity and the provision of quality care to all patients.

A gastroenterology nurse must be a combination of medical technician, educator, counsellor and advocate. Each of these skills and qualities contributes to comprehensive patient care, guaranteeing not only physical safety but also emotional and psychological well-being.

Continuing training and career development.

The medical world, with its frenetic pace of discovery and innovation, demands a constant commitment to continuing education. For gastroenterology nurses, this commitment is doubly essential. Not only does it guarantee quality care for patients, but it also offers opportunities for career development. Let's take a look at how continuing education can shape the career path of a nurse in this field.

- Specialised training modules:
  - These modules may cover specific areas such as advanced endoscopic techniques, the management of inflammatory bowel disease or new advances in nutritional therapy.
- Additional certifications :
  - These certifications, often offered by professional associations, validate expertise in particular areas of gastroenterology and strengthen the professional profile.
- Participation in conferences and workshops:
  - This enables nurses to interact with leading experts, discover the latest research and develop a professional network.
- Commitment to clinical research :
  - For those inclined towards research, taking part in clinical studies can open doors to research coordination or even advisory roles.

- Management and leadership training :
  - These courses prepare nurses for management roles, whether as team leaders, supervisors or even unit managers.
- Advanced specialisation :
  - Roles such as gastroenterology nurse practitioner may be envisaged, requiring advanced studies but offering greater clinical autonomy.
- Teaching :
  - With experience and training, some may choose to pass on their knowledge as clinical educators or instructors in nursing schools.
- Advisory roles :
  - In the field of medical devices or therapeutics, experienced nurses can be called on for their clinical expertise.

- Involvement in associations :
    - Active participation in professional associations can lead to leadership roles within these organisations.

The career path of a gastroenterology nurse is not limited to the patient's bed. With ongoing training, insatiable curiosity and a commitment to excellence, the possibilities are vast. Whether in the clinic, research, administration, teaching or consulting, every step of continuing education opens a new door, promising growth, satisfaction and impact in the vast field of gastroenterology.

Chapter 4
STANDARD PROCEDURES AND PROTOCOLS IN GASTROENTEROLOGY

Endoscopy : preparation, implementation and post-procedure monitoring.

Endoscopy is an essential procedure in gastroenterology, enabling certain areas of the digestive system to be viewed directly. For nurses, supporting patients before, during and after the examination is crucial to ensuring their safety and comfort. Let's take a closer look at the different stages of the procedure.

- Preparation for endoscopy :
    - **Prior consultation**: The nurse takes the patient's medical history, checks current medication and makes sure the patient understands the procedure.
    - **Fasting**: Depending on the type of endoscopy, the patient is generally asked to fast for a certain number of hours before the examination.
    - **Intestinal preparation**: For a colonoscopy, for example, it is essential that the colon is empty. The nurse provides clear instructions on the use of washing solutions or laxatives.
    - **Informed consent**: The nurse ensures that the patient has fully understood the procedure and its potential risks, and gives his/her consent for it to be carried out.

- Performing the endoscopy :
  - **Patient positioning** : The patient is placed in an appropriate position on the examination table, often on his or her side.
  - **Monitoring**: The nurse constantly monitors the patient's vital signs during the procedure, including blood pressure, heart rate and oxygen saturation.
  - **Administration of medication**: Sedatives or analgesics are often administered to ensure the patient's comfort. The nurse must ensure that they are administered correctly and monitor any reaction.
  - **Assisting the doctor**: The nurse assists the gastroenterologist by passing on the necessary instruments and helping to handle the endoscope if necessary.
- Post-procedure monitoring :
  - **Recovery**: After the procedure, the patient is taken to a recovery area where the nurse monitors vital signs and ensures that he or she wakes up properly from sedation.
  - **Detecting complications**: Although rare, complications such as bleeding or perforation can occur. Nurses must be vigilant and know how to identify these complications quickly.
  - **Post-procedure advice**: Before leaving, the nurse informs the patient about what to expect after the endoscopy, any side effects and when to resume a normal diet.
  - **Follow-up**: In some cases, a follow-up telephone call may be made to ensure that the patient is doing well and that there are no late complications.

Endoscopy is a common procedure in gastroenterology, but it requires meticulous attention at every stage to ensure the safety and well-being of the patient. Thanks to the expertise and care of the nurse, this procedure is made as comfortable and safe as possible, enabling crucial diagnostic information to be obtained or therapeutic interventions to be carried out.

Colonoscopy :
the procedure explained step by step.

Colonoscopy is an endoscopic procedure that enables the colon, or large intestine, to be examined in detail. It is an essential diagnostic tool for detecting conditions such as polyps, cancer or inflammation. Let's take a step-by-step look at the procedure.

- Reason for colonoscopy :
- Common reasons for recommending a colonoscopy include screening for colorectal cancer, assessing digestive symptoms (such as bleeding or abdominal pain) and monitoring pre-existing conditions such as inflammatory bowel disease.
- Preparation :
  - **Initial instructions**: Patients are given clear instructions regarding preparation, often a few weeks before the procedure.
  - **Special diet**: 1-2 days before the colonoscopy, it is generally advisable to follow a low-fibre diet and, the day before, a clear liquid diet.
  - **Bowel preparation**: In the evening before the examination (or sometimes the morning of the day of the examination), the patient takes a washing solution to completely clean the colon. This step is essential for obtaining clear images.

- The day of the procedure :
  - **Arrival and settling in**: After arriving at the clinic or hospital, the patient is placed in an examination gown. An intravenous catheter is often inserted to administer medication.
  - **Sedation**: Sedative drugs are usually administered to help the patient relax and remain comfortable during the procedure.
- The colonoscopy itself :
  - **Positioning**: The patient is usually positioned on his left side, with his legs slightly bent.
  - **Introducing the colonoscope**: A colonoscope, a flexible tube fitted with a camera, is gently inserted through the anus and advanced gently through the colon.
  - **Air insufflation**: Air or carbon dioxide is insufflated to inflate the colon and allow better visualisation.
  - **Examination**: The doctor examines the colon as the colonoscope is gradually withdrawn, looking for abnormalities such as polyps, tumours or inflammation. Biopsies may be taken if necessary.
  - **Polypectomy**: If polyps are detected, they can often be removed immediately using special instruments passed through the colonoscope.
- After the procedure :
  - **Recovery from sedation**: The patient is monitored in a recovery area until most of the effects of the sedation have worn off.
  - **Results**: The gastroenterologist usually discusses the initial results and any recommendations. If biopsies have been taken, it may be necessary to wait a few days for the final results.

- **Residual   gas** : Blowing in air can cause bloating or gas, which generally dissipates quickly.
- Post-procedure   recommendations :
  - Patients are generally asked to rest for the rest of the day.
  - Driving is not recommended for 24 hours after sedation, so it is often necessary to have someone accompany you home.

Colonoscopy is a safe and effective procedure when carried out by qualified professionals. It plays a crucial role in the prevention, diagnosis and treatment of various colon diseases.

Samples, biopsies and other routine tasks.

In gastroenterology, a variety of procedures are performed to diagnose or treat specific conditions. Let's explore some of the most common and their importance.

- Samples and biopsies:
  - **Gastric biopsy**: Used to assess inflammation, infections (such as *Helicobacter pylori*), or tumours of the stomach.
  - **Colon   biopsy**: Often performed during a colonoscopy, this is used to analyse polyps, diagnose inflammatory bowel disease or detect colorectal cancer.
  - **Liver   biopsy**: A sample of liver tissue is taken to assess liver diseases such as hepatitis, cirrhosis or tumours.
- Expansion:
  - **Oesophageal dilatation**: If the patient has a stenosis or narrowing of the oesophagus, a

34

special instrument can be used to gently dilate this area and improve the passage of food.
  - **Dilatation of the bile ducts**: In some cases, the ducts that carry bile can become narrowed. Dilatation improves the flow of bile.
- Polypectomy:
  - This is the removal of polyps, usually detected during a colonoscopy. This is an important preventive measure, as some polyps can develop into cancer.
- Endoscopic sphincterotomy:
  - This operation is performed to treat problems with the gallbladder or pancreas. It involves an incision in the sphincter of Oddi, the muscle that controls the flow of bile and pancreatic juices.
- Stenting:
  - If a duct or passage is blocked, for example in the case of a tumour, a stent (a small tube) can be inserted to keep the passage open.
- Endoscopic removal of tumours:
  - Some superficial tumours of the digestive tract can be removed endoscopically without the need for open surgery.
- Haemostasis:
  - Bleeding from the digestive tract can be treated by various endoscopic methods, such as injections, thermal coagulation or clips.
- Ligation of oesophageal   varices:
  - Oesophageal varices are dilated veins that can bleed. Ligation consists of placing an elastic band around the varicose vein to tie it off and stop the bleeding.

Each of these procedures requires specific preparation, technical skill and post-procedural monitoring. The role of the nurse is essential in ensuring patient safety, adequate preparation, smooth running of the procedure and appropriate follow-up.

Chapter 5
MANAGING ROUTINE CASES
IN GASTROENTEROLOGY

Inflammatory bowel diseases:
signs, symptoms and treatment.

Inflammatory bowel disease (IBD) is a group of disorders that cause prolonged inflammation of the digestive tract. The two main forms of IBD are Crohn's disease and ulcerative colitis. While these two diseases share common features, they affect different parts of the digestive tract.

- Crohn's disease :
- **Areas affected**: The entire digestive tract, from mouth to anus, can be affected. The inflammation is often deep and can affect all layers of the intestinal wall.
- **Signs and symptoms**: Abdominal pain, diarrhoea, weight loss, fever, fatigue, nausea, mouth ulcers, anal problems such as fissures, fistulas or abscesses.
- Ulcerative colitis :
- **Areas affected**: Only the large intestine (colon and rectum). The inflammation is generally more superficial, affecting the mucosa.
- **Signs and symptoms**: Bloody diarrhoea, abdominal pain and cramps, urge to have a bowel movement, fatigue, weight loss, fever.

Common risk factors :
- Family history
- Age (often diagnosed in young adults)
- Smoking (increases the risk of Crohn's disease and may protect against ulcerative colitis)

- Use of non-steroidal anti-inflammatory drugs (NSAIDs)

Treatments :
- Medicines :
    - **Aminosalicylates**: such as mesalazine or sulphasalazine, reduce inflammation.
    - **Corticosteroids**: such as prednisone, reduce inflammation and are used for acute flare-ups.
    - **Immunosuppressants**: such as azathioprine or mercaptopurine, reduce the activity of the immune system.
    - **Biological**: like infliximab or adalimumab, they specifically target certain substances involved in inflammation.
- Surgery:
    - **Crohn's disease**: In the event of complications or treatment-resistant disease, resection of the affected area may be necessary.
    - **Ulcerative colitis**: If medication is not effective, colectomy (removal of the colon) may be recommended.
- Other treatments:
    - **Nutrition**: Some patients may require nutritional supplements or a special diet, particularly during flare-ups.
    - **Probiotics**: Although research is still ongoing, certain strains of probiotics may help maintain remission.
- Symptom management:
    - Avoid common food triggers such as spicy, fatty or milky foods.
    - Manage stress, which can exacerbate symptoms.
    - Regular follow-up with a gastroenterologist to monitor the disease and adjust treatment.

The role of the gastroenterology nurse is crucial in the management of IBD patients. Whether educating patients about the disease, administering medication, monitoring side effects or providing emotional support, nurses play a pivotal role in patients' treatment pathways.

Liver and biliary tract disorders.

The liver is one of the largest and most complex organs in the body, playing a central role in digestion, detoxification and metabolism. The bile ducts are essential for transporting bile, a liquid produced by the liver to digest fats. A number of conditions can affect these essential structures.

- Hepatitis:
    - **Viral hepatitis**: Inflammation of the liver caused by one of the five hepatitis viruses (A, B, C, D, E). Symptoms include jaundice, fatigue, nausea and abdominal pain.
    - **Autoimmune hepatitis:** A chronic disease in which the immune system attacks the liver.
    - **Alcoholic hepatitis:** Inflammation and damage to the liver caused by excessive alcohol consumption.
- Cirrhosis:
    - Chronic scarring and liver dysfunction resulting from various conditions, such as chronic hepatitis or alcohol abuse.
- Liver cancer:
    - Can develop directly in the liver (hepatocellular carcinoma) or result from the spread of other cancers.
- Hepatic steatosis:
    - Accumulation of fat in liver cells, often associated with obesity, diabetes or excessive

alcohol consumption. Can progress to non-alcoholic steatohepatitis (NASH), a more serious form that can lead to cirrhosis.

- Primary biliary cholangitis (PBC):
  - An autoimmune disease which affects the small bile ducts inside the liver.
- Primary sclerosing   cholangitis (PSC):
  - Inflammation, scarring and obstruction of the bile ducts inside and outside the liver.
- Biliary lithiasis (gallstones):
  - Small stones formed in the gallbladder, which can block the bile ducts and cause severe pain.
- Cancer of the bile ducts (cholangiocarcinoma):
  - Malignant tumour that develops from the cells of the bile ducts.
- Infections:
  - **Hepatic abscess:** Accumulation of pus in the liver, usually caused by an infection.
  - **Acute   cholangitis**: Infection of the bile ducts, often due to a blockage.

Diagnosis and treatment:

Hepatobiliary disorders are diagnosed using a combination of blood tests, imaging studies (such as ultrasound, CT scan, MRI) and, in some cases, a liver biopsy.

Treatment varies according to the specific disease, ranging from drug interventions (such as antivirals for hepatitis) to surgery (for example, to remove gallstones or tumours). In severe cases, a liver transplant may be necessary.

As part of gastroenterology nursing care, patient education on prevention, symptom management, medication administration and monitoring for potential complications are essential. Nurses play a central role in supporting patients with hepatobiliary disorders, guiding their care pathway and ensuring optimal quality of life.

Gastritis, ulcers and other gastric disorders.

The stomach is a muscular cavity essential for digestion. However, because of its acidic environment, it is also vulnerable to a variety of ailments.

- Gastritis:
    - **Description**: Inflammation of the gastric mucosa.
    - **Causes**: Infections (often linked to *Helicobacter pylori*), alcohol abuse, long-term use of non-steroidal anti-inflammatory drugs (NSAIDs), stress, bile reflux, etc.
    - **Symptoms**: Abdominal pain or discomfort, nausea, vomiting, premature feeling of fullness.
- Gastroduodenal ulcers:
    - **Description**: Open lesions that form on the mucosa of the stomach (gastric ulcer) or duodenum (duodenal ulcer).
    - **Causes**: *H. pylori* infection, prolonged use of NSAIDs, genetic factors, smoking.
    - **Symptoms**: Burning or stabbing abdominal pain, nausea, acid reflux, weight loss.
- Gastroenteritis:
    - **Description**: Inflammation of the lining of the stomach and intestines.
    - **Causes**: Viral, bacterial or parasitic infections, food poisoning.
    - **Symptoms**: Diarrhoea, vomiting, abdominal cramps, fever, dehydration.
- Irritable stomach syndrome (nervous gastritis):
    - **Description**: Functional disorders with no detectable organic lesion.
    - **Causes**: Stress, inappropriate diet, hormonal disturbances.

- **Symptoms**: Abdominal pain, bloating, feeling of fullness, acid reflux.
- Gastric tumours:
  - **Description**: Abnormal growths of cells in the stomach, either benign (such as polyps) or malignant (gastric cancer).
  - **Causes**: Genetic factors, *H. pylori* infection, diet rich in salty and smoked foods, smoking, chronic atrophic gastritis.
  - **Symptoms**: Loss of appetite, weight loss, abdominal pain, nausea, vomiting, digestive bleeding.

Diagnosis and treatment:
The diagnosis of these gastric disorders is generally based on clinical symptoms, medical history, endoscopic examinations (gastroscopy), biopsies, blood tests and breath tests for *H. pylori*.
Treatment is tailored to the specific condition:
- Antibiotics to eradicate *H. pylori*.
- Proton pump inhibitors (PPIs) or H2 receptor antagonists to reduce gastric acidity.
- Antispasmodic medicines for functional disorders.
- Surgery in the event of ulcer complications or to remove tumours.
- Diet and nutritional advice to avoid triggers.

The role of the nurse is crucial in the management of gastric disorders. This includes educating the patient about taking medication, the importance of adhering to treatment, preventing complications and recommended dietary modifications. Nurses' ability to provide empathetic and educational care is essential in helping patients navigate these often painful and uncomfortable conditions.

Chapter 6
THE PATIENT-NURSE RELATIONSHIP: A BOND OF TRUST

Emotional challenges of care.

Nursing practice in the gastroenterology department is not just technical; it also has a considerable emotional dimension. The intimate and often complex nature of gastrointestinal conditions can make care emotionally demanding for both patient and healthcare professional.

- Patient vulnerability:
    - **Intimacy of examinations**: Procedures such as colonoscopy or endoscopy can be perceived as invasive and embarrassing for the patient.
    - **Stigma**: Conditions such as inflammatory bowel disease can cause embarrassing symptoms (diarrhoea, flatulence), which can lead to shame or embarrassment.
- Difficult to communicate:
    - **Announcement of serious diagnoses**: Informing a patient of a cancer or chronic illness can be emotionally distressing.
    - **Explaining complex procedures**: Simplifying medical concepts while ensuring patient understanding is a challenge.
- The nurse's emotional charge:
    - **Empathy vs over-investment**: Finding the balance between investing emotionally in the patient's well-being and maintaining a certain distance for the sake of your own mental health.

- **Burnout**: Repetitive tasks, stress and intense emotional situations can lead to burnout.
- Managing patient and family expectations:
  - **Hopes versus reality**: It is sometimes necessary to temper the hopes of patients or their families regarding treatment results or recovery times.
  - **Support at the end of life**: In the case of serious pathologies, supporting patients and their families at this stage is an emotionally heavy task.
- Working as part of a team:
  - **Interprofessional conflicts**: Differences of opinion about how a patient should be managed can lead to tension.
  - **Mutual emotional support**: It's crucial to be able to count on your colleagues for support, to share experiences or to decompress.
- Training and supervision:
  - **Lack of emotional training**: Most nursing training focuses on technical skills, sometimes leaving out the emotional aspect of care.
  - **Need for supervision**: Regular discussions with a supervisor or psychologist can help manage stress and emotions.

Adaptation strategies:
To meet these challenges, it is essential that nurses develop coping strategies:
- **Ongoing training**: Participate in training courses focusing on communication, emotional management or ethics.
- **Regular supervision**: Benefit from opportunities for exchange and reflection.
- **Well-being practices**: relaxation techniques, meditation, sports, hobbies, etc.

- **Support networks**: peer exchanges, discussion groups or psychological support.

Awareness and recognition of the emotional challenges associated with gastroenterology care are essential to ensure the well-being of professionals and optimal patient care.

Communication and patient education.

Communication is at the heart of gastroenterology nursing practice. It plays an essential role in the education, prevention, understanding and management of gastrointestinal disorders.

- Understanding the patient:
    - **Active listening**: Spending time listening to the patient helps us to understand their concerns, symptoms and expectations.
    - **Holistic assessment: looking** beyond physical symptoms to take account of the emotional, social and cultural dimensions of each individual.
- Passing on information:
    - **Simplification of medical terms**: Translate medical jargon into accessible language without compromising the accuracy of the information.
    - **Use of visual aids**: Diagrams, videos and mock-ups can make it easier to understand.
- Patient education:
    - **Disease self-management**: Training patients on how to manage their symptoms, take their medication and deal with emergencies.
    - **Preparing for procedures**: Clearly explaining the stages, risks and benefits of interventions.

- **Dietary advice**: Provide nutritional recommendations specific to each gastrointestinal condition.
- Managing emotions:
  - **Validation of feelings**: Recognising and validating the patient's emotions, whether fear, anxiety or frustration.
  - **Relaxation techniques**: Suggest techniques such as deep breathing or visualisation to help manage the stress associated with the illness or procedures.
- Involving the family:
  - **Joint education sessions**: Include the family or significant others in educational sessions so they can support the patient.
  - **Discussions on confidentiality**: Ensuring respect for privacy while recognising the crucial role of family members in care.
- Feedback and clarification:
  - **Checking comprehension**: Ask the patient to rephrase the information given to ensure that he or she understands it correctly.
  - **Willingness to ask questions**: Encourage the patient to ask questions, whether general or specific.
- Updating your knowledge:
  - **Ongoing training**: Nurses need regular training to keep up to date with new procedures, treatments and communication techniques.
  - **Sharing resources**: Offer patients brochures, links to reliable websites or recommendations for further reading.

Communication and education are two fundamental pillars of gastroenterology care. Effective communication builds trust, promotes adherence to treatment and improves clinical outcomes. Education empowers patients to play an active role in their own health, leading to informed choices and a better quality of life. Nurses, as intermediaries between the medical world and the patient, have a key responsibility in this area.

Managing difficult cases and delicate situations.

In a gastroenterology department, nurses are regularly confronted with complex situations, whether medical, emotional or relational. The ability to manage these cases and these delicate moments is essential to ensure the safety and well-being of the patient while preserving the professionalism of the nurse.

- Medically complex   cases:
    - **Multiple conditions**: Some patients may have several medical conditions at the same time, requiring special attention in the management of medicines and treatments.
    - **Adverse reactions**: The appearance of unexpected side effects or post-operative complications requires responsiveness and clinical expertise.
- Emotionally charged situations:
    - **Announcing a serious diagnosis**: Communicating bad news requires empathy, clarity and support.
    - **Managing bereavement**: Faced with a terminally ill patient or the death of a patient, it is essential to support the family and manage one's own emotions.
- Difficult relationships:
    - **Uncooperative   patients**: Some patients may refuse care or disagree with medical

recommendations. The key is to listen to them, clarify the issues and seek a compromise.

- **Demanding families**: Relatives can sometimes have unrealistic expectations or disagree with the medical team. The key is communication and setting clear limits.
- Ethical situations:
  - **Informed consent**: Ensuring that the patient fully understands all the implications of a procedure or treatment before giving consent.
  - **End of life and decisions to limit treatment**: These decisions, which are always complex, require a multidisciplinary approach and a profound respect for the wishes of the patient and their family.
- Challenges related to culture and language:
  - **Language barriers**: The use of interpreters or translation tools may be necessary to ensure clear communication.
  - **Respect for cultural beliefs**: Understanding and respecting the patient's cultural beliefs and practices can influence care.
- Managing stress and burnout:
  - **Recognising the signs**: Nurses need to be mindful of their own emotional and physical wellbeing, and recognise the signs of burnout.
  - **Professional support**: Seek help, whether through supervision, colleagues or professional resources.
- Patient feedback and complaints:
  - **Active listening**: Taking the time to listen to the patient's concerns or complaints.
  - **Proactive resolution**: Working with the medical team to address and rectify any issues raised.

Managing difficult cases and delicate situations is an intrinsic part of the gastroenterology nursing role. Adopting a patient-centred approach, combined with ongoing education, effective communication and professional support, enables us to navigate through these challenges with compassion, expertise and integrity.

Chapter 7
EMERGENCY SITUATIONS IN GASTROENTEROLOGY

Digestive haemorrhage: identification and intervention.

Digestive haemorrhage, whether upper or lower, is a medical emergency. Gastroenterology nurses play a crucial role in the rapid identification of such bleeding and the implementation of appropriate interventions.

- Definitions and classifications:
    - **Upper digestive haemorrhage (HDH):** Origin proximal to the ligament of Treitz, such as gastric or duodenal ulcers.
    - **Lower digestive haemorrhage (LDH):** Origin distal to the ligament of Treitz, often linked to disorders of the colon or rectum.
- Signs and symptoms:
    - **HDH**: Melena (black, tarry Feces), haematemesis (vomiting of blood), hypotension, tachycardia.
    - **HDB**: Rectorrhagia (bright red blood in the stools), bloody Feces, signs of shock if bleeding profusely.
- Initial assessment:
    - **Patient history**: Medications (anti-inflammatories, anticoagulants), history of ulcers or other gastrointestinal pathologies.
    - **Physical examination**: assessment of vital signs, abdominal examination, assessment of haemodynamic status.

- Initial treatment:
  - **Haemodynamic stabilisation**: Administration of solutions, blood transfusion if necessary.
  - **Insertion of a nasogastric tube**: In the case of HDH, to assess the presence and quantity of blood.
  - **Oxygen therapy**: Prevention of hypoxia.
- Diagnostic investigations:
  - **Endoscopy**: Used to identify the source of bleeding and, in many cases, to treat the lesion responsible.
  - **Colonoscopy**: Used in cases of suspected HDB.
  - **Angiography**: In certain situations where the source of bleeding is not clearly identified or if it persists.
- Therapeutic interventions:
  - **Endoscopic**: coagulation, clips, ligation of oesophageal varices.
  - **Medication:** Proton pump inhibitors to reduce gastric acidity, vasoconstrictors for oesophageal varices.
  - **Surgery**: If endoscopic and medicinal methods fail or are not possible.
- Post-intervention nursing care:
  - **Continuous monitoring**: vital signs, appearance of new bleeding.
  - **Patient education**: on medication, diet and the warning signs of a new haemorrhage.
  - **Emotional support**: A digestive haemorrhage is a traumatic experience for many patients.
- Prevention:
  - **Mucosa-protecting drugs**: For patients at risk of ulcers.

- **Avoid alcohol and irritating foods**: For patients with a history of digestive haemorrhage.
- **Vaccination**: against hepatitis B and C to reduce the risk of cirrhosis and oesophageal varices.

Digestive haemorrhage is a medical emergency requiring rapid and coordinated intervention. Thanks to their training and experience, nurses are on the front line in ensuring that patients are properly assessed, stabilised and cared for, while providing essential emotional and educational support.

Intestinal occlusions: signs, interventions and post-operative care.

Intestinal obstructions - mechanical or functional obstructions that prevent the normal passage of intestinal contents - are medical emergencies. They need to be identified and treated quickly to avoid serious complications. Nurses play a central role in this process.

- Definition and causes:
    - **Mechanical obstruction**: Due to a physical lesion preventing passage, such as a tumour, adhesions or a strangulated hernia.
    - **Ileus paralyticus**: cessation of intestinal contractions without mechanical obstruction, often due to surgery, infection or electrolyte imbalances.
- Signs and symptoms:
    - **Abdominal pain**: Often cramps and colic.
    - Abdominal distension.

- **Vomiting**: May be faecal in small bowel obstructions.
  - Absence of gas and Feces.
  - **Signs of dehydration**: dry mouth, pale complexion, oliguria.
- Initial assessment:
  - **Patient history:** surgical history, medication, associated symptoms.
  - **Physical examination**: Listen for bowel sounds (which may be hyperactive or absent), palpate the abdomen, look for signs of peritonitis.
- Diagnostic investigations:
  - **Abdominal X-rays**: To identify the location and cause of the obstruction.
  - **Abdominal scan**: For a more detailed view.
  - **Blood tests**: To check for electrolyte imbalances and other abnormalities.
- Initial treatment:
  - **Fasting**: To prevent further intestinal distension.
  - **Nasogastric tube**: To decompress the stomach and small intestine, relieving distension and vomiting.
  - **Rehydration:** Intravenous to correct dehydration and electrolyte imbalances.
- Therapeutic interventions:
  - **Surgery**: Necessary for mechanical occlusions that do not respond to conservative treatment, or in the presence of signs of strangulation or necrosis.
  - **Medical treatment**: In the case of paralytic ileus, management of the underlying causes, such as infection, and restoration of electrolyte balance.

- Post-operative nursing care:
    - **Vital monitoring**: Monitoring vital signs, pain and bowel sounds.
    - **Pain management**: Administration of analgesics as prescribed.
    - **Monitoring surgical wounds**: looking for signs of infection or complications.
    - **Nutritional support**: Initiation of a progressive diet once intestinal transit has resumed.
    - **Patient education**: on the signs of complications, wound care, diet and medication.
- Prevention of recurrences:
    - **Dietary advice**: Avoid foods that cause bloating or gas.
    - **Managing medication**: Certain medications can increase the risk of paralytic ileus.
    - **Physical rehabilitation**: Light exercise can help stimulate intestinal motility.

Bowel obstruction is a serious condition requiring rapid and appropriate intervention. Nursing management, from initial assessment through to post-operative care, is essential to ensure patient safety and well-being. Ongoing training and sharpened skills enable nurses to provide quality care and support patients at every stage of their recovery.

Other potential emergencies and their management.

In gastroenterology, in addition to haemorrhage and intestinal obstruction, a number of other emergencies can arise. Rapid intervention is crucial, and nursing care is central to the management of these situations.

- Gastrointestinal perforation:
  - **Signs**: Severe abdominal pain, rigid abdomen ("wooden belly"), fever, signs of shock.
  - **Management**: Fasting, gastric bypass for decompression, antibiotics, emergency surgery.
- Acute pancreatitis:
  - **Signs**: Intense abdominal pain radiating to the back, nausea, vomiting, abdominal distension.
  - **Management**: Fasting, analgesics, rehydration, treatment of electrolyte imbalances.
- Bleeding oesophageal varices:
  - **Signs**: Vomiting blood, melena, hypotension.
  - **Management**: Vasoconstrictive drugs, endoscopy for ligation or sclerotherapy, Blakemore catheter for uncontrolled haemorrhage.
- Acute appendicitis:
  - **Signs**: Right lower quadrant pain, fever, nausea.
  - **Management**: Emergency surgery to remove appendix, antibiotics.
- Acute cholecystitis:
  - **Signs**: Right upper quadrant pain, fever, nausea, vomiting.
  - **Management**: fasting, antibiotics, analgesics, cholecystectomy.
- Intestinal ischaemia:
  - **Signs**: Sudden and severe abdominal pain, bloody diarrhoea, distension.
  - **Management**: Revascularisation, surgery to remove necrotic segments, antibiotics.

- Fulminant hepatitis:
    - **Signs**: Jaundice, altered consciousness, bleeding.
    - **Management**: Intensive care unit monitoring, liver transplantation as a last resort.
- **Short bowel syndrome** (after extensive surgery) :
    - **Signs**: Diarrhoea, weight loss, nutritional deficiencies.
    - **Treatment**: Nutritional supplements, drugs to slow transit, possibly intestinal transplantation.

Each gastrointestinal emergency presents unique diagnostic and management challenges. Nurses must be well trained to recognise the early signs and symptoms of these conditions, initiate first aid and collaborate with a multidisciplinary team to ensure comprehensive management. Ongoing training and regular updating of knowledge are essential to ensure optimum care for patients in emergency situations.

Chapter 8
TEAMWORK: A NECESSARY SYNERGY

Collaboration with gastroenterologists.

Close collaboration between nurses and gastroenterologists is crucial to ensuring optimal patient care. This collaboration is not just limited to carrying out prescriptions, but extends to communication, care planning, patient education and much more.

- Initial assessment of the patient:
    - **Taking a history**: Nurses often take a detailed medical history of the patient and can identify key information for the gastroenterologist.
    - **Test preparation**: Helping to coordinate and prepare patients for endoscopic examinations or other investigations.
- Care planning:
    - **Discussion of complex cases**: exchanging information about the patient to develop an appropriate care plan.
    - **Participation in medical rounds**: updates on the patient's condition, symptoms and response to treatment.
- Procedures and treatments:
    - **Assistance during endoscopy**: patient preparation, follow-up during the procedure and post-operative monitoring.
    - **Administration of medication**: Monitor responses, side effects and communicate any concerns to the doctor.

- Patient education:
    - **Preparing for procedures**: explaining what to expect, answering questions.
    - **Managing medicines**: educating patients about dosage, side effects and potential interactions.
    - **Diet and nutrition**: offering advice on special diets, enteral or parenteral nutrition.
- Research and continuing education:
    - **Participation in clinical studies**: Nurses can help with data collection and patient monitoring.
    - **Joint training courses**: Attend seminars, conferences or workshops to keep up to date with the latest developments.
- Feedback and recommendations:
    - **Feedback**: Nurses are often the first to observe changes in the patient's condition and can recommend adjustments in care or treatment.
    - **Improving the quality of care**: Suggesting improvements based on daily observations or feedback from patients.

The collaboration between nurses and gastroenterologists is symbiotic, with each professional contributing their skills and expertise for the benefit of the patient. Open communication, mutual respect and a clear understanding of each other's roles are essential to ensure this fruitful collaboration and to provide the highest quality care.

The role of Caregivers and other paramedical staff.

In the context of gastroenterology, Caregivers and other paramedical staff play an essential role in ensuring overall

58

patient care. Their contribution goes well beyond basic assistance and is crucial to the smooth running of the department.

- Caregivers:
  - **Daily support**: Helping patients with daily activities such as washing, dressing and getting around.
  - **Vital signs**: Regular monitoring of vital signs and reporting of any abnormalities.
  - **Food and hydration**: Help patients to eat and drink, taking care to respect any special dietary requirements.
  - **Samples**: Collection of urine or Feces samples when necessary.
  - **Communication**: acting as an intermediary between the patient, the family and the medical team, and identifying patients' non-verbal needs.
- Physiotherapists:
  - **Post-operative rehabilitation**: Helping patients to recover after surgery or lengthy hospitalisation.
  - **Breathing exercises**: Essential for patients who have undergone abdominal surgery.
  - **Early mobilisation**: Encouraging mobility to prevent complications such as deep vein thrombosis.
- Dieticians:
  - **Nutritional assessment**: Analysing the patient's nutritional status to recommend an appropriate diet or supplements.
  - **Specific dietary advice**: For example, for patients suffering from inflammatory bowel disease or malabsorption.

- **Management of enteral and parenteral nutrition**: Monitor patients receiving specialised nutrition.
- Social workers:
  - **Emotional support**: Helping patients and their families to cope with illness, hospitalisation or stressful situations.
  - **Orientation**: Helping to plan hospital discharge, find community resources, organise rehabilitation or home care.
- Laboratory technicians:
  - **Analyses**: Carry out tests on blood, urine or Feces samples to aid diagnosis or follow-up.
  - **Reports**: Communicate abnormal results promptly for immediate action.

The paramedical staff, working closely with the nurses and doctors, guarantee holistic patient care. Each member brings a unique expertise, contributing to the richness and effectiveness of the care provided in gastroenterology. Recognition, ongoing training and good communication within this team are essential to optimising the quality of care.

Department meetings and continuity of care.

Continuity of care is a central pillar of modern medicine. For patients suffering from gastroenterological pathologies, which are often complex and require multidisciplinary management, ensuring continuity of care is crucial. Service meetings play a key role in ensuring that all the professionals involved are on the same wavelength and working together for the patient's well-being.

- Importance of department meetings:
    - **Exchanging information**: These enable the team to discuss complex cases, share relevant information and bring different perspectives to bear on a situation.
    - **Care planning**: defining the stages of care, organising procedures, allocating roles and responsibilities.
    - **Updating protocols**: Discussion of new guidelines and recent studies, and updating of care procedures and protocols accordingly.
- Key points discussed at the meetings:
    - **Case reviews**: Presentation of inpatients, their history, progress and challenges.
    - **Educational**: Presentation of new techniques, medicines or research relevant to the department.
    - **Organisational**: holiday planning, task allocation, resource and equipment management.
- Continuity of care and transition between teams:
    - **Effective communication**: Ensuring that key information is passed on between teams when changing departments or discharging patients.
    - **Medical records**: Ensuring they are up to date, accessible and understandable for all the professionals involved.
    - **Post-hospital follow-up**: Coordination with attending physicians, home care, rehabilitation services or any other external service.
- Involving patients and their families:
    - **Education**: Providing information about the disease, treatments, potential side-effects and what to do at home.
    - **Feedback**: Solicit feedback from patients and their relatives on their care experience, to constantly improve the quality of the service.

- **Discharge planning**: Ensuring a smooth transition for the patient to home or another institution.

Department meetings are not just administrative meetings. They are at the heart of the patient care strategy in gastroenterology. By ensuring fluid communication between professionals and actively involving patients and their families, they guarantee continuity of care, patient safety and, ultimately, clinical excellence.

Chapter 9
PREVENTION AND EDUCATION IN GASTROENTEROLOGY

Promoting healthy eating and adequate hydration.

In the field of gastroenterology, diet and hydration play a central role. A healthy diet and adequate hydration can not only prevent a large number of gastrointestinal diseases, but also optimise the healing process when a condition is already present. In this chapter, we look at the intimate relationship between the digestive tract and what we eat, and the importance of medical staff promoting good habits.

- The role of diet in gastroenterology:
    - **Disease prevention**: A balanced diet can reduce the risk of numerous pathologies such as gastritis, inflammatory bowel disease and certain cancers.
    - **Nutritional therapy**: In some cases, food can be used as a treatment, for example in the case of avoidance diets or specific diets for certain conditions.
- Main nutrients and their impact on the digestive system:
    - **Fibre**: Essential for colon health, it prevents constipation and reduces the risk of diverticulosis.
    - **Probiotics and prebiotics**: Beneficial for the intestinal flora, they can play a role in the treatment and prevention of irritable bowel syndrome.

- **Fats**: Consume in moderation, as too much can lead to digestive problems.
  - **Proteins**: Necessary for the repair and renewal of cells in the gastrointestinal mucosa.
- The importance of hydration:
  - **Role in digestion**: Water facilitates the passage of food through the digestive tract and helps to form Feces.
  - **Preventing constipation**: Sufficient hydration is essential to prevent constipation, a common problem in gastroenterology.
- Practical advice to promote healthy eating:
  - **Patient education**: Organise workshops or information sessions on nutrition.
  - **Working with dieticians**: They can provide specific advice tailored to each patient.
  - **Provision of resources**: Provide brochures, fact sheets or reference websites on food and gastroenterology.
- Challenges and obstacles to good nutrition:
  - **Access to quality food**: Not all patients have access to a healthy, balanced diet.
  - **Cultural factors**: Certain foods or eating habits may be rooted in the patient's culture.
  - **Comorbidities**: Certain illnesses or treatments can affect appetite or the ability to eat.

Promoting healthy eating and adequate hydration is a fundamental aspect of gastroenterology care. Through education and close collaboration with other health professionals, nurses can play an active role in improving patients' quality of life and preventing gastrointestinal diseases.

The importance of early detection gastrointestinal diseases.

The digestive tract is a complex organ that is the site of numerous pathologies, ranging from minor ailments to serious diseases that can be life-threatening. Against this backdrop, early detection of gastrointestinal diseases is of vital importance. Not only does it make it possible to intervene at a stage when the disease is more easily treatable, but also, in some cases, to prevent it from appearing in the first place.

- Prevention rather than cure:
    - **Reduced mortality**: Early detection of colorectal cancer, for example, can considerably reduce the risk of death by detecting and treating precancerous lesions.
    - **Less invasive and costly**: Treating a disease at an early stage can often avoid cumbersome, invasive and costly medical procedures.
- Commonly screened   gastrointestinal diseases:
    - **Colorectal cancer**: Screening tests such as Feces occult blood tests or colonoscopy can identify polyps or tumours at an early stage.
    - **Celiac   disease**: Blood tests can identify this autoimmune disease before severe symptoms appear.
    - **Viral hepatitis**: Regular screening can detect these infections before they lead to cirrhosis or liver cancer.
- Risk factors and target populations:
    - **Family history**: Certain gastrointestinal diseases have a hereditary component, justifying early screening of individuals at risk.
    - **Age**: Diseases such as colorectal cancer are more common after a certain age, hence the

need for regular screening for the populations concerned.

- **Specific exposures**: For example, people who have been exposed to certain infections, drugs or chemicals may require targeted screening.
- Awareness-raising and education:
  - **Information campaigns**: Raising public awareness of the importance of screening through media campaigns, workshops and brochures.
  - **Medical consultations**: Use every visit to the doctor as an opportunity to assess the need for screening.
- The challenges of screening:
  - **Patient compliance**: Some patients may be reluctant to undergo screening tests because of fear, denial or lack of knowledge.
  - **Access to care**: In certain regions or populations, access to screening tests may be limited due to financial or geographical constraints.

Early detection of gastrointestinal diseases is a crucial step towards effective prevention, treatment and management. With the right awareness of the risks and close collaboration between healthcare professionals and patients, it is possible to significantly reduce the burden of these diseases on society.

Raising awareness of diseases linked to smoking and alcohol.

Smoking and excessive alcohol consumption are among the leading preventable causes of morbidity and mortality worldwide. In addition to their well-known effects on the lungs and liver, these two risk factors also have major repercussions on the gastrointestinal system. Raising awareness of these dangers is essential to prevent and limit the damage caused.

- Smoking and the gastrointestinal system:
  - **Oesophageal and stomach   c a n c e r**: Smoking significantly increases the risk of developing these types of cancer.
  - **Inflammatory bowel   disease**: Smoking is associated with a more severe course of Crohn's disease and may influence the response to treatment.
  - **Gastro-oesophageal   reflux disease**: Smoking weakens the sphincter of the oesophagus, increasing the risk of acid reflux.
- Alcohol and its effects on the digestive tract:
  - **Cirrhosis and liver cancer**: Alcohol is one of the main causes of cirrhosis and also increases the risk of liver cancer.
  - **Alcoholic pancreatitis**: Excessive consumption can inflame the pancreas, causing pain and dysfunction.
  - **Alcoholic gastritis**: Alcohol can irritate the lining of the stomach, causing inflammation.
- Populations at risk:
  - **Young adults**: Young people are often exposed to social pressure to drink alcohol and start smoking.
  - **Patients with a family history**: Individuals with a family history of alcohol- or smoking-related conditions should be particularly vigilant.
- Awareness-raising strategies:
  - **Education from an early age**: Introduce prevention programmes in schools to raise awareness right from the start.

- **Advertising campaigns**: Using the media to broadcast powerful awareness-raising messages showing the consequences of smoking and alcohol abuse.
- **Targeted consultations**: Offer awareness-raising and weaning sessions in health centres.
- Multi-disciplinary collaboration:
  - **Working with addictology specialists**: Addictology specialists play a key role in the overall care of patients.
  - **Intervention by psychologists**: To understand and treat the underlying reasons for addiction.
- The challenges of raising awareness:
  - **Stigmatisation**: Patients may feel judged or ashamed, which can be a barrier to seeking help.
  - **Cultural and social beliefs**: In some cultures, the consumption of alcohol or tobacco is deeply rooted, making raising awareness more complex.

Smoking and excessive alcohol consumption have devastating effects on the gastrointestinal system, among other body systems. Active, ongoing awareness-raising is the key to reducing the prevalence of these harmful habits and their consequences. By combining the efforts of healthcare professionals, educators and the media, it is possible to make a significant difference and save many lives.

Chapter 10
REFLECTIONS AND TESTIMONIALS: EVERYDAY LIFE SEEN FROM THE INSIDE

Testimonials from experienced nurses: challenges, successes and memorable moments.

Testimonial 1 - Léa, 15 years of service
"When I started my career in gastroenterology, I was impressed by the complexity of the procedures and equipment. The biggest challenge was managing to remain calm and reassuring to patients during endoscopy procedures, while managing my own anxiety. But with time, experience and the support of my team, I developed a comfort level. The day I was able to manage a digestive haemorrhage emergency on my own was a turning point in my career, showing me that I was far more capable than I imagined."

Testimonial 2 - Omar, 20 years of service
"One of my most memorable moments was caring for a young patient with Crohn's disease. Seeing her daily struggle reminded me why I had chosen this profession. Helping patients manage chronic conditions is a constant reminder of the fragility of life and the importance of our role. When she came back, years later, just to say thank you, it reaffirmed that our work is about much more than medical care; it's about building relationships."

Testimonial 3 - Fatima, 18 years of service
"Working in gastroenterology presents constant challenges, from keeping abreast of the latest technological advances to dealing with tricky situations.

But one of the achievements I'm most proud of is mentoring young nurses. Passing on my knowledge to them and seeing their passion and determination to develop is extremely gratifying. Every time a nurse I've trained succeeds, I feel it's my own success."

Testimonial 4 - Benjamin, 25 years of service
"One of the major challenges I've encountered over the years is communicating with patients from different cultures and languages. I had one patient who spoke very little of our language and was very anxious about his colonoscopy. With patience, gestures and the help of a translator, we managed to put him at ease. After the procedure, he drew a heart on a piece of paper and gave it to me. It reminded me that compassion is a universal language."

The testimonials from gastroenterology nurses highlight the human side of the profession, the challenges they face, but also the moments of success and fulfilment. Despite the technical complexity of the speciality, it is the human interaction, the ability to make a difference to patients' lives, that remains at the heart of their experience.

Lessons learned over the years.

Over the course of a career in gastroenterology, nurses accumulate a wealth of experiences and lessons that shape not only their professional practice, but also their personal outlook. Here are a few key lessons, often mentioned by professionals with years of experience in the field:
- **The importance of active listening**: Patients, in all their vulnerability, need to be heard. Active listening

not only leads to better diagnosis and care, but also to a relationship of trust between nurse and patient.

- **Adaptability is key**: Medicine is constantly evolving, as are technologies and protocols. Nurses must be prepared to learn and adapt throughout their career to provide the best possible care.
- **Caring above all**: It's not just about mastering a technique or protocol. Caring, empathy and compassion are central to the nurse's role. These qualities can make all the difference to a patient's experience.
- **Collaboration is essential**: Teamwork with doctors, Caregivers and other healthcare professionals is crucial. Open and respectful communication is the key to ensuring smooth and effective care.
- **Prevention is as important as treatment**: Educating patients about prevention, whether in terms of diet, lifestyle or risk awareness, is often as important as the treatment itself.
- **The importance of self-care**: Nurses are often so focused on their patients' well-being that they forget about their own. Taking time for oneself, recognising one's own limitations and seeking support when necessary are essential for a sustainable and fulfilling career.
- **Every patient is unique**: although symptoms may be similar, each patient is an individual with his or her own experiences, concerns and needs. An individualised approach to care is essential.
- **The importance of continuing education**: Gastroenterology is a constantly evolving field. A commitment to continuing education ensures that nurses remain at the cutting edge of the best practices and treatments.
- **Patience is a virtue**: Whether it's waiting for results, managing a patient's fears or mastering a new skill, patience is often one of a nurse's most valuable tools.

- **The power of gratitude**: A simple thank you from a patient, an acknowledgement from a family or even a moment of personal satisfaction after a difficult day - these small moments of gratitude remind us of the profound reason why we chose this profession.

Beyond technical skills and medical knowledge, it is often the intangible lessons, learned through human interaction and the challenges of everyday life, that resonate most deeply with gastroenterology nurses. These lessons not only shape their careers, but also enrich their lives immeasurably.

Advice for newcomers to the department.

Starting out in a gastroenterology department, or any medical department, can be both exciting and intimidating. It's a world rich in learning, human experience and technical challenges. Here is some advice for those taking their first steps in this speciality:

- **Embrace lifelong learning**: Don't expect to know everything from the start. Medicine is a constantly evolving field, and gastroenterology is no exception. Be curious and open to new knowledge.
- **Ask for help when you need it**: Nobody expects you to know everything. If you're unsure or have questions, ask your more experienced colleagues for advice. It's a sign of professionalism, not weakness.
- **Build strong relationships with your team**: Teamwork is crucial in this business. Get to know your colleagues, understand their strengths and weaknesses, and build a strong team spirit.
- **Be patient and empathetic with yourself**: As with any new role, there will be difficult days. It's important

to remember that every mistake is a learning opportunity.

- **Familiarise yourself with the equipment**: Gastroenterology uses a lot of specific equipment. Take the time to get to know them, learn how to use them and, above all, understand their importance for the patient.
- **Prioritise communication**: Clear communication with patients, families and the team is essential. This helps to prevent errors, educate effectively and build trust.
- **Take part in training courses and workshops**: Take advantage of all the continuing education opportunities on offer, whether seminars, workshops or readings.
- **Keep a global perspective**: Don't get lost in the details at the expense of the big picture. Each patient is an individual with his or her own history, concerns and needs.
- **Develop relaxation routines**: Stress is inherent in this profession. Find techniques that allow you to relax and decompress after a day's work, whether it's meditation, sport, reading or any other hobby.
- **Stay passionate**: Always remember why you chose this career. It is this passion that will guide you through the challenges and help you find satisfaction in your work.

The early stages of a career in gastroenterology can seem daunting, but with the right attitude, support and a willingness to learn, it can be one of the most rewarding journeys of your professional life. Every day brings new discoveries, meaningful interactions and opportunities to make a positive impact on patients' lives.

Chapter 11
PHARMACOLOGY
IN GASTROENTEROLOGY

Commonly used medicines and their indications.

Gastroenterology covers a wide range of conditions, and many medicines are used to prevent, treat or manage these diseases. Here is a non-exhaustive list of medicines commonly used in this field, with their main indications:

- Antacids and proton pump inhibitors (PPIs) :
  - Examples: Omeprazole (Mopral®), Esomeprazole (Nexium®), Lansoprazole (Lanzor®)
  - Indications: Gastroesophageal reflux disease (GERD), gastritis, gastric and duodenal ulcers, Zollinger-Ellison syndrome.
- Antispasmodics :
  - Examples: Phloroglucinol (Spasfon®), Dicyclomine (Bentyl®)
  - Indications: Treatment of pain associated with intestinal spasms, irritable bowel syndrome.
- Prokinetics :
  - Examples: Metoclopramide (Primpéran®), Domperidone (Motilium®)
  - Indications: Nausea and vomiting, gastroparesis, gastro-oesophageal reflux.
- Coating agents :
  - Examples: Sucralfate (Ulcar®)
  - Indications: Gastritis, gastric and duodenal ulcers.

- Antidiarrhoeals :
    - Examples: Loperamide (Imodium®), Racecadotril (Tiorfan®)
    - Indications : Acute or chronic diarrhoea.
- Laxatives :
    - Examples: Bisacodyl (Dulcolax®), Macrogol (Forlax®), Lactulose (Duphalac®)
    - Indications: Constipation.
- Antiemetics :
    - Examples: Ondansetron (Zophren®), Granisetron (Kytril®)
    - Indications: Nausea and vomiting, including that induced by chemotherapy.
- Anti-inflammatory agents for the digestive tract :
    - Examples: Mesalazine (Pentasa®), Budesonide (Entocort®)
    - Indications: Crohn's disease, haemorrhagic rectocolitis.
- Specific antibiotics for the digestive tract :
    - Examples: Rifaximin (Xifaxan®)
    - Indications: Irritable bowel syndrome with predominant diarrhoea, hepatic encephalopathy.
- Antiviral agents :
    - Examples: Entecavir (Baraclude®), Tenofovir (Viread®)
    - Indications: Chronic hepatitis B.
- Hepatic protectors :
    - Examples: Ursodeoxycholic acid (Delursan®)
    - Indications: Primary biliary cholangitis, biliary cirrhosis.
- Probiotics :
    - Examples: Lactobacillus, Bifidobacterium
    - Indications: Maintenance of intestinal flora, prevention and treatment of antibiotic-associated diarrhoea.

This list is just an overview of the medicines used in gastroenterology. It is essential for nurses to understand not only the indications, but also the interactions, side-effects and contra-indications of these medicines to ensure that patients are treated safely.

Drug interactions to watch out for.

Drug interactions are changes in the efficacy or toxicity of a drug when administered with another drug, food or even drink. In gastroenterology, given the wide range of drugs used, it is essential to monitor these interactions closely to ensure patient safety. Here are some common and important drug interactions in the field:

- Proton pump inhibitors (PPIs) :
    - **Clopidogrel**: PPIs may reduce the efficacy of clopidogrel, increasing the risk of cardiovascular events.
    - **Azole antifungals**: PPIs can reduce the absorption of azole antifungals such as ketoconazole and itraconazole.
- Antispasmodics :
    - **Anticholinergics**: Combining antispasmodics with other anticholinergic drugs may increase the risk of side effects such as dry mouth, constipation and confusion.
- Prokinetics (e.g. Metoclopramide) :
    - **Antipsychotics**: Increased risk of extrapyramidal effects when metoclopramide and antipsychotics are taken together.
    - **Digoxin**: Metoclopramide may increase the absorption of digoxin, thereby increasing the risk of toxicity.

- **Mesalazine** (used in inflammatory bowel disease) :
  - **Azathioprine and 6-mercaptopurine**: Combination may increase the risk of myelosuppression.
- Rifaximin :
  - **Oral anticoagulants**: Rifaximin may increase the levels of oral anticoagulants, increasing the risk of bleeding.
- Stimulant laxatives (e.g. Bisacodyl) :
  - **Diuretics and corticosteroids**: Increased risk of electrolyte imbalance and dehydration.
- Anti-inflammatory agents for the digestive tract (such as budesonide):
  - **CYP3A4 inhibitors** (e.g. ketoconazole, erythromycin): Increased risk of systemic toxicity due to budesonide.
- Ursodeoxycholic acid :
  - **Clofibrate, oral contraceptives and oestrogens**: These drugs can increase hepatic cholesterol secretion, reducing the effectiveness of ursodeoxycholic acid.

These interactions are just a few of the many possible in gastroenterology. Monitoring drug interactions is a responsibility shared between doctors, nurses and pharmacists. Open and continuous communication between these professionals is crucial to preventing undesirable interactions and ensuring optimal patient care.

Administration and supervision side effects.

The way in which a drug is administered can greatly affect its effectiveness, while monitoring for side effects is crucial to ensuring patient safety. In gastroenterology, as in other medical specialities, knowledge of both these aspects is vital.

Administration of medicines :
- **Route of administration**: Some medicines can be administered orally, intravenously, rectally or subcutaneously. The choice of route depends on the patient's condition, the nature of the drug and its mechanism of action.
- **Administration times**: Some drugs, such as PPIs, are more effective when administered before meals to maximise their effect on reducing gastric acidity.
- **Food interactions**: Some medicines can interact with food, either by reducing their absorption or by increasing the risk of side effects. For example, taking alcohol with certain medicines can aggravate liver damage or increase the risk of bleeding.

Monitoring side effects :
- Common gastrointestinal effects :
  - Diarrhoea, constipation, nausea, vomiting.
  - Abdominal pain, bloating.
  - Changes in the colour or consistency of Feces.
- Systemic effects :
  - Skin rashes, itching.
  - Dizziness, headaches, confusion.
  - Changes in kidney or liver function, which can be assessed by blood tests.
- Allergic reactions :
  - Hives, oedema, breathing difficulties.
  - In the event of a severe allergic reaction, rapid intervention is required.
- **Monitoring vital signs**: Some medicines can affect blood pressure, heart rate or breathing.
- **Long-term effects**: Some medicines, when used long-term, can have cumulative side effects or

delayed effects. It is essential to have regular appointments to monitor these effects.

- **Monitoring drug interactions**: Combining several drugs can lead to new side effects or reinforce the undesirable effects of each drug.
- **Patient education**: Patients need to be informed about the potential side effects of the medicines they are taking. Open communication will enable patients to report any adverse effects quickly, thereby improving their safety.

Proper administration of medicines and careful monitoring of side effects are essential for the safe and effective management of gastroenterology patients. Nurses play a key role in this, acting as the first line of defence in identifying and managing drug side effects.

Chapter 12
SPECIFIC POST-OPERATIVE CARE

Pain management
and post-surgical complications.

Pain and post-surgical complications are common concerns in gastroenterology, given the invasive nature of many procedures. Nurses, along with the entire medical team, play an essential role in managing, preventing and alleviating these problems.

1. Pain management:
Pain assessment :
- Use of pain scales, such as the visual analogue scale, to quantify pain.
- Take into account factors such as the location, duration, intensity and type of pain (stabbing, burning, etc.).

Pharmacological interventions :
- Non-opioid analgesics: paracetamol, non-steroidal anti-inflammatory drugs (NSAIDs), etc.
- Opioid analgesics: morphine, oxycodone, etc. Use with caution.
- Adjuvant medication: antispasmodics, tricyclic antidepressants or anti-epileptics for neuropathic pain.

Non-pharmacological interventions :
- Relaxation and meditation techniques.
- Application of heat or cold to the painful area.
- Complementary therapies such as acupuncture and massage therapy.

2. Post-surgical complications:

Infections :
- Monitoring for signs of infection such as fever, redness, purulent oozing and oedema.
- Administration of prophylactic or therapeutic antibiotics as indicated.

Bleeding :
- Regular monitoring of dressings and drains to detect excessive bleeding.
- Monitoring blood parameters such as haemoglobin and haematocrit.
- Administration of blood products as required.

Postoperative Ileus (slowing or stopping of intestinal transit) :
- Monitoring bowel sounds.
- Encouraging early mobilisation.
- Nutrition management, starting with clear liquids and then progressing cautiously to solid food.

Pulmonary complications (such as atelectasis or pneumonia) :
- Encourage deep breathing exercises and coughing.
- Use of an incentive spirometer.
- Early mobilisation of the patient.

Venous thromboembolism :
- Use of compression stockings or pneumatic compression devices.
- Early mobilisation.
- Medication prophylaxis with anticoagulants if indicated.

Wound-related complications :
- Watch for signs of dehiscence (separation of wound edges) or evisceration (protrusion of internal organs through the wound).
- Keep the wound clean and dry.

The management of pain and post-surgical complications is a delicate balance requiring constant monitoring and rapid intervention. Gastroenterology nurses must work closely with surgeons, anaesthetists and other members of the healthcare team to ensure patients' comfort and safety throughout their recovery.

Monitoring signs of complications.

Monitoring is a key element in the management of gastroenterology patients. Early identification of signs of potential complications can make the difference between a favourable outcome and clinical deterioration. Here is an overview of the main signs to look out for:

1. Post-endoscopic complications :
   - **Perforation**: Intense abdominal pain, distension, fever, absence of gas or Feces.
   - **Bleeding**: Presence of blood in vomit or Feces, melena (black, tarry stools).

2. Post-surgical complications :
   - **Infections**: Fever, redness, heat or oozing from the surgical wound, chills.
   - **Bleeding**: Anaemia, pallor, tachycardia, hypotension, active bleeding from the wound.
   - **Venous thromboembolism**: Pain, redness, swelling of a limb, shortness of breath, chest pain.

3. Complications associated with the disease :
   - **Intestinal obstruction**: abdominal distension, vomiting, constipation, absence of gas.
   - **Digestive haemorrhage**: vomiting of blood, melena, paleness, drop in blood pressure.
   - **Peritonitis**: Intense abdominal pain, rigidity of the abdomen, fever.

4. Drug complications :
- **Hepatotoxicity**: jaundice (yellowing of the skin or eyes), dark urine, fatigue, abdominal pain.
- **Allergic reactions**: skin rash, itching, swelling of the face or throat, breathing difficulties.

5. Dehydration and electrolyte imbalances :
- **Dehydration**: Intense thirst, dry mouth, dark urine, weakness, dizziness.
- **Electrolyte imbalances**: muscle cramps, weakness, palpitations, oedema.

6. Complications of hepatic steatosis :
- **Cirrhosis**: jaundice, ascites (accumulation of fluid in the abdomen), easy bleeding, oedema.

7. Acute pancreatitis :
- Intense abdominal pain, nausea, vomiting, fever, tachycardia.

Active, regular monitoring of vital signs, biological parameters and the patient's clinical symptoms is essential. Communication is also essential: patients should be encouraged to report any unusual or worrying symptoms. Early intervention in the event of complications can often improve outcomes and minimise damage. Nurses, on the front line of this surveillance, play a central role in the detection and management of complications in gastroenterology.

Rehabilitation and patient education after surgery.

After gastroenterology surgery, rehabilitation and patient education are essential to promote rapid recovery, minimise the risk of complications and ensure a better quality of life in the long term. Here is a detailed overview of this post-intervention phase:

1. Physical rehabilitation :
   - **Early mobilisation**: Encouraging the patient to get up, walk and move around as soon as authorised by the medical team to avoid complications associated with immobility, such as venous thrombosis.
   - **Breathing exercises**: Teaching and encouraging techniques such as deep breathing and the use of an incentive spirometer to prevent pulmonary complications.
   - **Progressive feeding**: Start with clear liquids, then progress to more solid foods, taking into account the specific recommendations linked to the intervention.

2. Pain management :
   - **Medication**: Inform the patient about how and how often to take analgesics, and about any side effects.
   - **Non-pharmacological methods**: Encourage techniques such as relaxation, meditation or the application of heat to relieve pain.

3. Wound care :
   - **Maintenance**: Educate the patient on the daily cleaning of the wound, how to recognise the signs of infection, and how to change a dressing if necessary.
   - **Monitoring**: Report signs of complications, such as excessive bleeding, separation of wound edges or release of unusual fluids.

4. Drug education :
   - **Instructions**: Ensure a clear understanding of the medication regime, doses, timings and duration of treatment.
   - **Side-effects**: Information on common side-effects and what to do in the event of an adverse reaction.

5. Dietary advice :
- **Adapted diet**: Providing recommendations on foods to be favoured or avoided depending on the nature of the operation and the patient's specific condition.
- **Hydration**: Stress the importance of adequate hydration and, if necessary, give instructions on the amount and type of fluids to consume.

6. Activities and restrictions :
- **Resuming activities**: Give instructions for gradually resuming daily activities, exercise and work.
- **Restrictions**: Information on activities to be avoided, such as lifting heavy objects, during the recovery period.

7. Medical follow-up :
- **Appointments**: Remind patients of the importance of follow-up visits to monitor healing and detect any complications.
- **Communication**: Encourage patients to communicate openly with the medical team if they have any concerns or unexpected symptoms.

The post-operative period is a crucial time that requires special attention. Appropriate rehabilitation and education not only support recovery, but also enhance the patient's autonomy, enabling them to play an active part in their own recovery process.

Chapter 13
PSYCHOLOGICAL ASPECTS IN GASTROENTEROLOGY

Managing anxiety related to procedures and diagnostics.

Fear of the unknown, fear of the results, or simply the discomfort associated with a medical procedure can be a major source of anxiety for gastroenterology patients. Managing this anxiety is essential to ensure the patient's well-being and the success of the procedure.

1. Education and information :
   - **Clear explanation**: Describe the procedure or diagnosis in simple terms, explaining why it is necessary and how it will be carried out.
   - **Visual material**: Use brochures, videos or diagrams to help illustrate and clarify the process.
   - **Questions and answers**: Encourage the patient to ask questions and answer them with patience and empathy.

2. Psychological preparation :
   - **Relaxation techniques**: teaching patients methods such as deep breathing, meditation and visualisation.
   - **Emotional support**: offering active listening, validating the patient's feelings and providing a safe space to express concerns.

3. The right environment :
   - **Soothing atmosphere**: Ensure a calm environment, with subdued lighting, soft music or soothing sounds if possible.

- **Confidentiality**: guaranteeing a private space for consultations, examinations and sensitive discussions.

4. Support :
  - **Presence of a relative**: If the patient so wishes, a member of their family or a friend may accompany them to appointments or operations.
  - **Peer support**: Encourage patients to join support groups where they can share their experiences and hear those of others.

5. Pharmacological strategies :
  - **Anxiolytics**: In some cases, medication may be prescribed to reduce anxiety before a procedure. It is essential to discuss the benefits, risks and possible side effects.

6. Post-procedure feedback :
  - **Open discussion**: After the procedure, take the time to talk to the patient, answer their questions and debrief about what went well or what was difficult.
  - **Improvement strategies**: Solicit feedback from patients on their experience to optimise management during future operations.

7. Access to psychological support :
  - **Psychotherapy**: If necessary, refer the patient to a therapist or psychologist specialising in supporting patients with chronic illnesses or facing medical interventions.
  - **Counselling**: Offer sessions with a specialist health adviser to help manage anxiety and concerns about diagnosis or treatment.

Recognising and addressing patient anxiety is fundamental to holistic care. By understanding and addressing their fears, healthcare professionals can greatly improve the patient experience and, consequently, clinical outcomes.

Psychological support for chronic diseases.

The management of chronic illnesses such as Crohn's disease, ulcerative colitis or cirrhosis of the liver requires a holistic approach, integrating not only physical care but also psychological support. Faced with a chronic diagnosis, patients can experience a myriad of emotions, ranging from denial and anger to grief and acceptance. It is therefore essential to provide appropriate psychological support to improve quality of life and disease management.

1. Recognising emotional needs :
   - **Regular assessment**: Use standardised screening tools to regularly assess patients' mood and emotional well-being.
   - **Open dialogue**: Encourage patients to express their concerns, fears and feelings about their illness.

2. Individual therapy :
   - **Psychotherapy**: Cognitive-behavioural therapy, acceptance and commitment therapy or other methods may be useful for managing the stress, anxiety and depression associated with a chronic illness.
   - **Tip**: Counselling sessions can help patients navigate the day-to-day challenges of managing their disease.

3. Support groups :
   - **Exchanging experiences**: Enabling patients to share their experiences, tips and advice with others in the same situation.

- **Involving specialists**: Invite experts to discuss specific subjects, such as nutrition, medication or pain management.

4. Workshops and training :
- **Stress management**: Offer workshops on meditation, mindfulness or yoga to help manage stress and anxiety.
- **Disease education**: Providing information about the disease, available treatments and the latest research, to help patients feel informed and in control.

5. Family intervention :
- **Family support**: Offer information and support sessions for family members to help them understand the disease and support their loved one effectively.
- **Family therapy**: In some cases, family therapy can be beneficial in addressing the specific tensions or challenges associated with the illness.

6. Access to resources :
- **Documentation**: Provide brochures, books and other written material on the disease and its management.
- **Referral to specialists**: Referring patients to psychologists, psychiatrists or other specialists according to their specific needs.

7. Adherence to treatment :
- **Follow-up support**: Helping patients to understand the importance of following their treatment and providing support to overcome potential barriers to adherence.
- **Regular feedback**: Encourage patients to express their feelings about their treatment and discuss any changes or adjustments that may be necessary.

Effective and appropriate psychological support can greatly improve the quality of life of patients with chronic gastroenterological conditions. A holistic approach that takes into account both the physiological and emotional needs of the patient is essential to ensure the best possible outcome.

Relationships with patients' families and their role in care.

A patient's family plays a vital role in the patient's care. In gastroenterology, where diagnoses and treatments can be complex and sometimes chronic, collaboration with families is essential to comprehensive care. This relationship, based on trust, empathy and respect, not only promotes the patient's recovery, but also strengthens the therapeutic partnership.

1. Understanding and information :
   * **Educating families**: informing them about the disease, treatments and procedures, so that they can provide informed support to the patient.
   * **Information sessions**: Organise regular meetings to answer families' questions and keep them informed of developments.

2. Active participation in care :
   * **Relay role**: The family can play an essential role in relaying information between the medical team and the patient, particularly if the patient is unable to communicate.
   * **Home support**: Ensuring a smooth transition when the patient returns home, by training families in basic care or the administration of medication.

3. Emotional management :
- **Psychological support**: Recognising that families may also feel anxiety or stress when faced with the illness of a loved one, and offering them resources to help them cope.
- **Space for expression**: Providing a safe environment where families can share their concerns, fears and hopes.

4. Medical decisions :
- **Joint decision-making**: Include the family in medical decisions, especially if the patient is unable to decide for themselves, in order to respect the patient's wishes and values.
- **Advance care planning**: Encourage families to discuss advance directives with the patient, to be prepared for any eventuality.

5. Respect and cultural integration :
- **Understanding family values**: Every family has its own beliefs, values and traditions. It is important to recognise these and incorporate them into the care plan.
- **Interpreting services**: Ensuring that families who speak other languages or have specific cultural needs have the resources they need to understand and be understood.

6. Support at the end of life :
- **Palliative support**: Working closely with families as the patient approaches the end of life, ensuring that they are supported, informed and involved in decisions.

Working closely with families in the gastroenterology department not only makes the family a partner in care, but also enhances the patient's overall well-being. The nurse-family relationship should be based on mutual respect, trust and open communication, ensuring the best possible care for the patient.

Chapter 14
ETHICS AND DEONTOLOGY
IN GASTROENTEROLOGY

Respect for patient autonomy
and informed consent.

In the vast world of medicine, and in gastroenterology in particular, respect for patient autonomy is a cornerstone of ethical practice. This autonomy means that each individual has the inalienable right to make decisions about his or her own health. These decisions, however, must be based on a full and clear understanding of the proposed medical interventions, their implications and the potential associated risks. This is where the principle of informed consent comes in.

Informed consent is not just an administrative formality or a signature on a document. It is a dynamic process, an ongoing conversation between the patient and the medical team. This dialogue enables the patient to fully understand the nature of the procedure or treatment, its potential benefits, the associated risks, and the alternatives available.

In gastroenterology, for example, before an endoscopy or colonoscopy, it is vital that the patient understands not only the details of the procedure itself, but also the reasons why it is recommended, any complications and alternative treatment options. This ensures that the patient is not passively subjected to the treatment, but is an active and informed participant.

The medical team, for its part, is responsible not only for providing all the relevant information, but also for ensuring that the patient has understood it. This may require rephrasing, illustrating with examples, or using visual aids. Patients should feel free to ask questions, express concerns or reservations, and take the time they need to reflect on their decision.

But beyond the information aspect, respect for patient autonomy and informed consent encompass a profoundly human and emotional dimension. It means recognising the uniqueness of each individual, his or her concerns, fears, aspirations and values. In some cases, particularly when faced with decisions with far-reaching consequences, patients may need psychological support or guidance to help them make an informed choice.

In gastroenterology, as in all medical disciplines, respect for patient autonomy and informed consent are more than just legal or ethical obligations. They represent the quintessence of respectful, patient-centred medicine, where every intervention is the fruit of a shared, fully informed decision.

Managing common ethical dilemmas.

Medicine, with its complex range of situations and decisions, is fertile ground for ethical dilemmas. In gastroenterology, as in other medical specialities, healthcare professionals are often faced with delicate choices that challenge their sense of morality and ethics.

1. Autonomy versus medical benefits :
One of the most common ethical tensions is that between respect for patient autonomy and the practitioner's desire to act in the patient's best medical interests. A patient may, for example, refuse a colonoscopy despite worrying clinical signs. In such cases, the medical team must weigh the

patient's right to refuse treatment against the potential benefits of the procedure.

2. Full disclosure versus patient protection :
How much information should be given to the patient? Sometimes too much information can cause unnecessary anxiety, but not providing enough could compromise informed consent. It's a question of striking a balance between full disclosure and protecting the patient's emotional well-being.

3. Managing unrealistic expectations :
Some patients may have unrealistic expectations about the outcome of a treatment or procedure. The gastroenterologist is then faced with the dilemma of trying to meet the patient's wishes or setting limits based on medical and ethical criteria.

4. Conflicts of interest :
Modern medicine, with its technological advances and links with industry, can present situations where financial or research interests can conflict with patient welfare. It is crucial to identify these conflicts and manage them transparently.

5. End-of-life decisions :
In gastroenterology, complex decisions can arise, particularly in the case of patients with terminal illnesses such as certain cancers. The question of whether to prolong treatment, introduce palliative measures or discontinue certain treatments can be a source of profound ethical dilemmas.

6. Confidentiality :
Respect for privacy and confidentiality is essential, but situations may arise where the public interest or the welfare of others may justify disclosure of information, such as in the case of contagious diseases.

Faced with these dilemmas, it is essential for gastroenterologists and the medical team as a whole to have a solid ethical framework, often based on principles such as autonomy, beneficence, non-maleficence and justice. In addition, the use of hospital ethics committees can provide a valuable external perspective for navigating these sensitive issues.

At the heart of these dilemmas is always the patient's well-being, and it is with empathy, respect and integrity that these ethical challenges must be addressed.

Confidentiality and patient rights.

Confidentiality is an essential pillar of the doctor-patient relationship. It is the guarantee of the trust that patients place in their carers, in the knowledge that the sensitive information they share will only be used within the strict framework of their medical care. In gastroenterology, as in other specialities, confidentiality is of particular importance.

Confidentiality: a fundamental right
The right to confidentiality is enshrined in many medical codes of ethics around the world. This right stipulates that all information relating to the patient, whether it concerns their medical history, examinations, treatments or any other aspect of their care, must remain strictly confidential. In gastroenterology, this may include detailed information about a patient's digestive health, procedures such as colonoscopies, or diagnoses such as inflammatory bowel disease.
Limits and exceptions to confidentiality

While confidentiality is a fundamental principle, it is not absolute. There are certain situations where disclosure of information may be justified:

- **Patient consent**: If a patient explicitly agrees to certain information being shared, for example with other specialists for a second opinion, confidentiality can be waived.
- **Overriding interest**: In rare situations, disclosure of medical information may be necessary to protect public health or prevent imminent danger to the patient or others.
- **Legal obligations**: Certain countries or jurisdictions may require the disclosure of medical information in specific circumstances, such as the detection of certain contagious diseases.

Patients' rights

In addition to confidentiality, patients have a number of rights:
- **Access to information**: Every patient has the right to access his or her medical file, to obtain a copy of it and to request clarification of any element it contains.
- **Correcting data**: If a patient believes that any information in their file is incorrect, they have the right to ask for it to be corrected.
- **Informed consent**: No medical procedure can be carried out without the free and informed consent of the patient. This means that the patient must be fully informed of the implications, risks and benefits of the procedure.
- **Refusal of treatment**: All patients have the right to refuse treatment or an operation, even if this goes against medical recommendations.

Confidentiality and respect for patients' rights are more than just legal or ethical obligations. They embody the essence of respectful, patient-centred medical practice, where each individual is recognised and treated with dignity, respect and kindness. In gastroenterology, as in all medical fields, these principles guide every interaction, every diagnosis and every treatment, ensuring quality care that respects the fundamental rights of every patient.

CHAPTER 15
THE IMPORTANCE OF
CLINICAL RESEARCH

Participation in clinical trials and testing.

Medical research is constantly evolving, seeking better ways to treat, diagnose or even prevent disease. In gastroenterology, this is particularly relevant given the complexity and diversity of disorders of the digestive system. Clinical studies and therapeutic trials are essential steps in translating scientific discoveries into beneficial clinical interventions for patients.

Why take part in clinical trials?
- **Medical advances**: Clinical trials are used to evaluate new treatments, new therapeutic approaches or new diagnostic techniques.
- **Access to innovative treatments**: Participants may have access to new treatments that are not yet widely available.
- **Contribution to science**: Taking part in a clinical trial means contributing to the advancement of medical science and, potentially, helping future patients.

Important considerations for nurses
- **Patient education**: Nurses play a key role in informing patients about the progress of trials and the potential benefits and risks.
- **Increased monitoring**: Patients taking part in trials may need to be monitored more closely for possible side effects.

- **Reporting and documentation**: Accuracy is crucial. Nurses must ensure that all results, observations and interventions are meticulously recorded.

Informed consent
Any patient potentially eligible for a clinical trial must give informed consent. This means that they must be fully informed of the objectives of the study, the procedures involved, the potential benefits and risks, and the right to withdraw from the study at any time without prejudice to their care.

Ethics of clinical trials
Clinical trials are governed by strict ethical standards to ensure the safety and well-being of participants. All trials must be approved by an independent ethics committee before they begin. In addition, the confidentiality of participants must be preserved at all times.

Prospects for patients
While some patients may benefit directly from taking part in a clinical trial, others may see no direct benefit. Nevertheless, contributing to medical research is in itself rewarding.

Clinical studies and therapeutic trials in gastroenterology offer the opportunity to advance medical science and provide innovative solutions to the challenges posed by digestive diseases. Nurses, as key players in patient management, have an essential role to play in ensuring that these studies run smoothly, by providing effective communication, careful monitoring and accurate documentation.

The nurse as link between patients and research.

Nurses occupy a unique position in the world of healthcare, because of their proximity to and constant interaction with patients. In addition to their clinical responsibilities, nurses play a crucial role as a bridge between the patient and the vast field of medical research. In the speciality of gastroenterology, this role is all the more important given the rapid development of knowledge and treatments in this field.

Information facilitator
- **Demystifying research**: Nurses have the ability to translate complex medical jargon into terms that are more accessible to patients, helping them to understand the issues, objectives and processes involved in clinical studies.
- **Discussion of options**: The clinician may present the patient with the various studies or clinical trials available, explaining the potential benefits and associated risks.

Assessment of suitability
The nurse, who knows the patient well, is able to assess whether the patient is a good candidate for a specific clinical study. This assessment takes into account the patient's general health, medical history and other criteria specific to each study.

Emotional support
The prospect of taking part in a clinical study can be a source of anxiety for some patients. The nurse's reassuring presence can provide emotional support, listen to patients' concerns and answer their questions.

Rigorous monitoring
During the study, the nurse plays an essential role in patient follow-up. They ensure that the protocols are followed, monitor and document any side effects, and guarantee that any intervention or medication is administered correctly.

Promoting research
Through their testimony and commitment, nurses can encourage other patients to consider taking part in clinical studies, thereby reinforcing the importance of research in advancing gastroenterology care.

Continuing education
To remain an effective link between the patient and research, nurses need to engage in ongoing training. This enables them to keep abreast of the latest advances in gastroenterology, as well as new research methodologies.

The gastroenterology nurse is not only a care provider, but also a true ambassador for research. They educate, inform, support and guide patients through the sometimes complex world of medical research. Thanks to their unique position, nurses actively contribute to bringing science closer to the people it aims to help, making patients active partners in the development of medicine.

Recent advances from research in gastroenterology.

The field of gastroenterology is constantly evolving, driven by relentless scientific discoveries. These advances offer new perspectives on treatment and improve the quality of life of patients suffering from gastrointestinal disorders. Here's a look at some of the notable advances that have emerged from recent research in this speciality:

Intestinal microbiota and health

- **Microbiome studies**: Detailed studies of the gut microbiome have highlighted its crucial role in many aspects of our health, from inflammatory bowel disease to diabetes and even certain neurological disorders.
- **Microbiota-based therapies**: The use of faecal microbiota transplants to treat recurrent *Clostridium difficile* infections is an example of an innovative therapy resulting from this research.

Advanced endoscopy technologies

- **Endoscopic capsules**: These small cameras, swallowed like a pill, make it possible to view areas of the digestive system that were previously inaccessible without surgery.
- **Confocal endoscopy**: This technology enables microscopic images of the intestinal mucosa to be obtained during endoscopy, providing early detection of pathological changes.

Treatment of inflammatory bowel disease (IBD)

- **Biologically targeted therapies**: Treatments such as anti-TNF or JAK inhibitors have revolutionised the management of IBD, offering relief to many patients resistant to traditional treatments.
- **Studies on diet**: Research has highlighted the importance of diet in the management of IBD, leading to new dietary recommendations.

Early detection and treatment of gastrointestinal cancers

- **Advanced screening techniques**: The use of artificial intelligence in endoscopy enables more accurate detection of precancerous lesions.
- **Targeted therapies and immunotherapies**: These new approaches have shown promising results in the treatment of certain advanced gastrointestinal cancers.

The role of diet in gastrointestinal disorders
- **FODMAP diets**: Research has shown the effectiveness of low FODMAP diets in managing the symptoms of irritable bowel syndrome.
- **The role of gluten**: Beyond coeliac disease, non-celiac gluten sensitivity is an area of active research, aimed at better understanding and treating this disorder.

Mechanisms of gastrointestinal pain
Research has shed light on the complex mechanisms of pain in conditions such as irritable bowel syndrome, paving the way for new therapeutic strategies.

These advances represent just the tip of the iceberg in a constantly evolving field. Gastroenterology research continues to provide innovative solutions to medical challenges, offering hope and improved quality of life to patients around the world.

Chapter 16
HEALTH AND WELL-BEING THE NURSE

Managing stress and avoid burnout.

The nursing profession, with its responsibilities and demands, can be particularly trying. In gastroenterology, nurses have to deal with complex, emotionally-charged and potentially stressful situations on a daily basis. Managing stress and preventing burnout are therefore essential to ensuring the quality of care and well-being of nurses.

Recognising the signs of stress and burnout
The first step to managing stress effectively is to recognise the signs. Persistent fatigue, irritability, sleep problems, reduced motivation, feelings of disillusionment or inefficiency can all be indicators of chronic stress or the onset of burnout.
Implementing adaptation strategies
  - **Prioritisation and delegation**: Knowing how to determine the urgency of situations and delegating when possible can reduce the workload and the feeling of being overwhelmed.
  - **Taking breaks**: Taking regular short breaks during the day helps to recharge your batteries and reduce tension. These moments can be used to stretch, breathe deeply or simply relax for a few minutes.
  - **Managing your time**: Organising your day well, setting achievable goals and avoiding procrastination can reduce stress.
Taking care of yourself
  - **Balanced diet**: Proper nutrition is essential for maintaining energy and concentration.

- **Physical activity**: Even moderate exercise can help relieve stress, improve mood and build resilience.
- **Quality sleep**: A good night's sleep is crucial to recovering from a demanding day.

Seeking support

- **Supervision and mentoring**: Talking to a supervisor or mentor can provide valuable advice, a different perspective and emotional support.
- **Support from colleagues**: Sharing your experiences with colleagues can offer relief, as they can understand and empathise with the challenges you face.
- **Seek advice if necessary**: If the stress becomes too overwhelming, it may be beneficial to consult a health professional, whether a psychologist, counsellor or other specialist.

Personal development and training

- **Meditation and relaxation techniques**: Mindfulness, meditation and other relaxation techniques can help manage stress.
- **Ongoing training**: Acquiring new skills can boost confidence and reduce feelings of insecurity.

Setting limits

It's crucial to recognise your limits and know when to say no or ask for help. This avoids spreading yourself too thin and allows you to concentrate on the essential tasks.

The well-being of gastroenterology nurses is essential not only for themselves, but also for providing quality care to patients. Recognising, anticipating and managing stress and burnout can ensure a long, fulfilling and mutually beneficial career.

Relaxation and self-care techniques.

The medical world is often demanding, particularly for nurses working in specialities such as gastroenterology. To continue providing quality care while maintaining their own well-being, it is essential for nurses to adopt relaxation and self-care techniques. These methods can help to reduce stress, prevent burnout and improve quality of life.

Deep breathing
One of the simplest but most effective methods of inducing relaxation is deep breathing. It allows you to :
- Reduce heart rate
- Reduce muscle tension
- Promoting concentration
- To practise, simply sit or lie down comfortably, close your eyes, breathe in slowly through your nose, fill your lungs completely and then exhale slowly through your mouth.

Meditation and mindfulness
These techniques have gained in popularity because of their many advantages, including :
- Stress reduction
- Improved concentration
- Promoting a sense of calm and inner peace
- Whether it's guided meditation, body scanning or simply observing your breathing, a few minutes a day can make a big difference.

Physical exercise
Physical activity is an excellent way of :
- Relieving stress
- Improving mood through the release of endorphins
- Maintaining good general health

- Whether it's brisk walking, yoga, swimming or any other form of exercise, the important thing is to find an activity you enjoy and do it regularly.

Visualisation techniques
Visualisation involves imagining a place or situation that evokes relaxation. It allows you to :
- Take your mind off everyday concerns
- Cultivating positive feelings
- This technique can be particularly useful before a stressful procedure or after a difficult day.

Journaling
Writing regularly can help to :
- Clarifying your thoughts
- Recognising and dealing with emotions
- Finding solutions to problems
- You don't need to write at length, just a few lines about how you felt during the day.

Body care
Treatments such as massages, hot baths or aromatherapy can :
- Reduce muscle tension
- Improve blood circulation
- Promoting general relaxation

Disconnection
In a constantly connected world, it's beneficial to take time away from screens, be they computers, phones or television. This allows you to :
- Reducing mental stimulation
- Promoting better quality of sleep
- Reconnecting with the immediate environment

Ultimately, each nurse must find the techniques that suit him or her best. The important thing is to recognise the importance of self-care and to take regular time out to recharge. Mental and emotional health is just as crucial as physical health, especially in professions as demanding as gastroenterology nursing.

Support among colleagues and the importance of the professional network.

In the complex and demanding world of medicine, and particularly in specialities such as gastroenterology, professional relationships are of paramount importance. Solidarity between colleagues and the development of a strong professional network are key to guaranteeing quality care, while preserving the mental health and well-being of carers.

Colleague support: an unsuspected strength
Collaboration between nurses, doctors, Caregivers and other healthcare professionals is much more than a simple working dynamic. It creates a mutually supportive environment where :

- **Sharing experiences**: nurses can share practical advice, tips and techniques for dealing with complex situations.
- **Mutual understanding**: Who better than a colleague to understand the day-to-day challenges, stressful situations and emotions that certain clinical cases can generate?
- **Emotional support**: In difficult times, having a colleague to talk to, who can offer a sympathetic ear, is invaluable.
- **Collaboration in care**: Patients often benefit from multidisciplinary care. Fluid communication between the various parties involved ensures continuity of care and better case management.

The professional network: broadening your horizons

Having a solid professional network goes far beyond relationships between colleagues in the same establishment. It involves :

- **Continuing education**: Conferences, seminars and training courses are excellent opportunities to meet professionals from other institutions, exchange practices and learn about the latest advances.
- **Inter-hospital exchanges**: Collaboration between different hospitals or clinics can enrich each other's practices and improve patient care.
- **Career opportunities**: An expanded professional network can open doors to work, research and teaching opportunities.
- **Research and innovation**: Nurses who want to get involved in research can find mentors, partners or collaborators through their network.

Fostering a supportive environment

It is crucial for healthcare establishments to recognise the importance of support between colleagues and the creation of professional networks. This can take the form of :

- Time for debriefing after complex situations.
- Setting up discussion or supervision groups.
- Encouraging participation in professional events and training courses.
- Promoting a culture of mutual support and respect.

A well-supported nurse is a professional who is more fulfilled, more competent and therefore better able to provide quality care. In a speciality as demanding as gastroenterology, this professional solidarity is not only beneficial for nurses, it is also essential for ensuring the well-being of patients.

Chapter 17
TECHNOLOGY AND INNOVATION
IN GASTROENTEROLOGY

Appliances and
state-of-the-art diagnostic tools.

In the dynamic world of medicine, gastroenterology stands out for the rapid adoption of advanced technologies, enabling a better understanding, accurate diagnosis and optimised therapeutic intervention for gastrointestinal diseases. These technological advances, combined with the clinical expertise of our professionals, have revolutionised patient care.

The high-definition endoscope
Endoscopy, which explores the inside of the digestive tract, has benefited from a number of innovations. The introduction of high-definition imaging provides a much improved view of the mucous membranes, making it possible to detect tiny lesions or subtle changes.

Confocal endomicroscopy
This technique combines traditional endoscopy with confocal microscopy, enabling microscopic images of tissue to be obtained in real time. This offers unprecedented diagnostic accuracy, particularly for differentiating benign from malignant tumours.

Capsule enteroscopy
Also known as a "pillcam", this is literally a mini-camera inserted into a capsule that the patient swallows. It passes through the digestive system, sending high-definition

images of the small intestine, a region that is difficult to access by other means.

Ultrasound endoscopy (EUS)
This technique combines endoscopy and ultrasound, providing detailed images of the walls of the digestive organs and adjacent structures. It is an invaluable tool for assessing tumours, cysts and other abnormalities.

High-resolution manometry
Used to assess oesophageal function, this technology provides a detailed representation of oesophageal contractions, helping to diagnose conditions such as achalasia or diffuse oesophageal spasm.

The SmartPill
This is an ingested capsule that measures pressure, pH and temperature throughout the gastrointestinal tract. It is particularly useful for assessing gastric emptying and intestinal motility.

Hydrogen meter
This device measures the amount of hydrogen exhaled, helping to diagnose conditions such as lactose intolerance or excessive bacterial growth in the small intestine.

The importance of training and updating
With the emergence of these cutting-edge technologies, ongoing training for nurses and doctors is essential. Not only do they need to understand how these devices work, but also how to interpret the data they provide, while ensuring patient safety and comfort.
In conclusion, gastroenterology is at the forefront of technological adoption in medicine, offering ever more precise and effective diagnostic and therapeutic tools. These advances, combined with the expertise of

healthcare professionals, promise better quality care and improved outcomes for patients.

Telemedicine and its role in remote consultation.

In an increasingly connected world, telemedicine has emerged as an innovative solution to overcome some of the traditional barriers to accessing healthcare. Particularly in gastroenterology, telemedicine has revolutionised the way patients interact with their doctors and receive medical advice.

What is telemedicine?
Telemedicine refers to the provision of healthcare services at a distance using information and communication technologies. This can include medical consultations via videoconferencing, remote patient monitoring, patient education and even some forms of telemonitoring.

The benefits of telemedicine in gastroenterology
- **Improved access**: Telemedicine eliminates geographical constraints, giving patients living in remote areas access to gastroenterology specialists.
- **Time savings**: Patients no longer need to travel or wait in waiting rooms, reducing the time spent on consultations.
- **Continuity of care**: Patients can easily follow up after an operation or treatment, which is essential for chronic diseases such as Crohn's disease or ulcerative colitis.
- **Prevention**: Early access to a doctor can help detect and treat problems at an early stage.

Challenges and considerations
- **Security and confidentiality**: Ensuring the security of patient information is paramount. Telemedicine platforms must comply with data protection regulations.
- **Quality of care**: It is essential that telemedicine does not compromise the quality of care. Although remote consultation is practical, it cannot always replace a face-to-face assessment.
- **Technology and infrastructure**: Telemedicine requires appropriate equipment and a stable Internet connection. Not all patients have access to these resources.
- **Training and adaptation**: Healthcare professionals need to be trained to use telemedicine tools effectively and to adapt their communication skills to this format.

The future of telemedicine in gastroenterology
With the proliferation of connected devices and the emphasis on patient-centred care, it is likely that telemedicine will continue to play an increasing role in gastroenterology. This may include the integration of telemedicine into telemonitoring, with devices such as camera pills or tracking sensors enabling real-time monitoring of patients.

Telemedicine in gastroenterology offers a unique opportunity to widen access to care, promote prevention and improve patients' quality of life. Its success will depend on widespread adoption by healthcare professionals, acceptance by patients, and the introduction of appropriate regulations and protocols.

Future innovations
and their potential impact on practice.

Gastroenterology, like many other medical fields, is constantly evolving. Technological and scientific innovations are transforming the way healthcare professionals diagnose, treat and manage gastrointestinal conditions. In this context, it is essential for all professionals to understand and anticipate the impact of these innovations on daily practice.

The miniaturisation of diagnostic tools
With the advent of nanotechnology and micro-devices, diagnostic tools have become smaller and more efficient. Pill cameras, for example, can now navigate the digestive system to provide detailed images without the need for invasive intervention.
Impact: Less stress and discomfort for patients. Reduced need for anaesthesia and invasive procedures.

Gene therapy and personalised medicine
The growing understanding of the human genome and the specific genetic markers associated with certain gastrointestinal diseases means that targeted treatments can now be envisaged.
Impact: More effective treatments, fewer side effects and a better understanding of disease progression.

Artificial intelligence (AI) in gastroenterology
AI, combined with medical imaging, can help to quickly and accurately identify abnormalities, such as polyps during a colonoscopy.
Impact: Faster diagnosis, fewer human errors and improved quality of care.

Microbiomes and targeted therapy
Research into the intestinal microbiome has highlighted its role in many gastrointestinal disorders. Therapies using probiotics or even microbiota transplants are currently being studied.

Impact: Innovative therapeutic approaches that could revolutionise the treatment of diseases such as irritable bowel syndrome and Crohn's disease.

Virtual training and augmented reality
Augmented reality and virtual reality could be used to train doctors and nurses in complex procedures, offering an immersive learning experience.

Impact: Better preparation of professionals, reducing the risk of errors and improving patient safety.

Gastroenterology is on the cusp of a major transformation thanks to these innovations. However, despite the undeniable benefits of these advances, it is essential to approach these new technologies with caution, ensuring that medical ethics and patient safety remain at the heart of any adoption. These innovations, while promising, will also require ongoing training to ensure their optimal integration into everyday clinical practice.

Chapter 18
RARE DISEASES
AND COMPLEX CASES
IN GASTROENTEROLOGY

Presentation less common illnesses.

Gastroenterology is a vast field that encompasses a wide range of diseases, from the most common to the rarest. While conditions such as gastro-oesophageal reflux disease (GERD) and Crohn's disease are relatively well known, there are other less common conditions that are just as important for healthcare professionals and patients to understand.

1. Chronic intestinal pseudo-obstruction (CIPO)
This condition is characterised by symptoms of intestinal obstruction with no obvious mechanical cause. Patients often experience abdominal pain, nausea and distension, without any real blockage.
Main symptoms: Abdominal pain, vomiting, severe constipation.
Treatment: Therapeutic approaches may include prokinetic drugs, adapted diet and, in extreme cases, surgery.

2. Ogilvie syndrome
This is an acute dilatation of the colon in the absence of mechanical obstruction. It is often associated with surgery, infection or medication.
Main symptoms: Abdominal distension, pain, constipation.

117

Treatment: Treatment is generally based on correcting the underlying cause, stopping the drugs responsible and, in some cases, decompressing the colon.

3. Diverticular disease of the small intestine
Unlike colonic diverticulosis, this condition is rare and involves small diverticula that form in the small intestine.
Main symptoms: Abdominal pain, diarrhoea, bleeding.
Management: Antibiotics to treat associated infections, a specific diet and, in some cases, surgery may be necessary.

4. Zollinger-Ellison syndrome
This rare syndrome is caused by tumours in the pancreas or duodenum that secrete too much gastrin, leading to excessive production of gastric acid.
Main symptoms: Stomach or duodenal ulcers, diarrhoea, gastro-oesophageal reflux.
Management: Proton pump inhibitors to reduce acid secretion and surgery to remove tumours.

5. Primary sclerosing cholangitis
This is a liver condition in which the bile ducts become inflamed and scarred. It is often associated with ulcerative colitis.
Main symptoms: Jaundice, itching, abdominal pain.
Treatment: Medication to treat inflammation, surgery to open blocked bile ducts and, in advanced cases, a liver transplant.

Although less common, these diseases represent a challenge for healthcare professionals because of their complex diagnosis and multidimensional management. In-depth knowledge of these diseases, coupled with close collaboration between gastroenterologists, surgeons, radiologists and other specialists, is crucial to providing patients with the best possible care.

Management of atypical cases and differential diagnosis.

In the practice of gastroenterology, as in other medical fields, it is not uncommon to encounter atypical cases. These situations can challenge the initial diagnosis, requiring a methodical approach to establish an accurate and effective diagnosis. Differential diagnosis plays a crucial role here, enabling clinicians to distinguish between several conditions that present similar symptoms.

1. Importance of differential diagnosis
The differential diagnosis is a cornerstone of clinical medicine. It is a list of possible conditions that the clinician establishes on the basis of the patient's symptoms and clinical signs. In gastroenterology, symptoms are often non-specific, making the initial diagnosis tricky. Abdominal pain, for example, can have dozens of possible causes.

2. Dealing with common but misleading symptoms
- **Abdominal pain**: Causes may include ulcers, gallstones, appendicitis, diverticulitis and many more. The location, nature and associated symptoms can help narrow down the list of differential diagnoses.
- **Diarrhoea**: Is it infectious, inflammatory, functional like IBS (Irritable Bowel Syndrome), or perhaps due to malabsorption like coeliac disease?
- **Dysphagia (difficulty swallowing)** : Is it a mechanical problem such as cancer or stenosis, or is it due to a motor disorder such as achalasia?

3. Use of diagnostic tools
Once the clinician has established a list of possible diagnoses, various diagnostic tools, such as endoscopy, ultrasound scans, blood tests and biopsies, can be used to confirm or exclude specific conditions.

4. Challenges posed by atypical presentations

Atypical cases do not follow the manual. A patient may present with symptoms that seem contradictory or are discreet. In these situations, careful listening to the patient, a detailed clinical history and close monitoring are essential.

5. Importance of consultation and collaboration

When dealing with complex or atypical cases, collaboration with colleagues and even consultation with specialists from other disciplines can be invaluable. In addition, a review of the patient's medical history, medication and recent travel can often provide crucial clues.

Managing atypical cases in gastroenterology requires a combination of sharp clinical skills, in-depth knowledge of the pathology and a holistic approach to the patient. Whilst recognising the limits of their own expertise, gastroenterologists must be prepared to seek advice from colleagues and rethink their initial assumptions to ensure the best possible management of the patient.

Collaboration with other specialities for complex cases.

Gastroenterology, although specialised, does not operate in a silo. It is closely interconnected with other medical disciplines, mainly because the gastrointestinal system interacts with almost every other system in the body. In complex cases where symptoms go beyond the typical gastrointestinal disorder, collaboration with other specialists is not only beneficial but often essential to ensure holistic patient management.

1. Common connections in gastroenterology
- **General surgeons**: For procedures such as bowel resections, gallbladder removal or operations on the liver and pancreas.
- **Radiologists**: For in-depth imaging, such as MRI, CT scan or endoscopic ultrasound.
- **Rheumatologists**: Many inflammatory bowel diseases, such as Crohn's disease, can have extra-intestinal manifestations, including joints.
- **Dermatologists**: Certain gastrointestinal conditions, such as coeliac disease, can manifest themselves through skin symptoms.
- **Endocrinologists**: The liver plays an essential role in regulating metabolism, and disorders such as fatty liver are often linked to endocrine disorders, particularly diabetes.

2. Communication and coordination

Medical teams need to work closely together, sharing their knowledge and expertise to establish an accurate diagnosis and treatment plan for the patient. This is facilitated by multidisciplinary meetings where cases are discussed, medical images reviewed and treatment decisions made jointly.

3. Navigating intersections

Gastrointestinal disease can often be a symptom or aggravating factor of another underlying condition. For example, heart failure can cause liver congestion. In these cases, the ability to work in tandem with other specialists, such as cardiologists, is crucial.

4. Education and training

Continuing education and the exchange of information between specialities are essential. Workshops, conferences and joint meetings enable gastroenterologists and their colleagues from other disciplines to keep abreast of the latest advances in each field.

Medicine is an interconnected field. By recognising the value of multidisciplinary collaboration, healthcare professionals can ensure a more comprehensive approach to care, addressing the varied and complex needs of their patients. In the world of gastroenterology, this collaboration is particularly relevant, as the gastrointestinal system is at the heart of many systemic interactions.

Chapter 19
PATIENT TRANSITION :
THE HOSPITAL WARD AT HOME

Discharge planning and care coordination.

Discharge planning is a crucial stage in a patient's care. It ensures that patients receive the care and support they need to manage their illness or convalescence safely at home or in another care setting. In gastroenterology, where conditions can range from simple indigestion to serious illness requiring surgery, discharge planning is multi-dimensional and needs to be carefully co-ordinated.

1. Patient assessment
Before discharge is planned, a thorough assessment of the patient is required. This assessment includes :
- **Current medical condition**: Is it stable? What are the potential risks?
- **Medication requirements** : What medication does the patient need to take? How often?
- **Ability to self-manage**: Is the patient able to look after themselves at home? Does he need assistance?
- **Home environment**: Is the patient's home adapted to their current medical needs? Are there any potential obstacles or hazards?

2. Planning and coordination
- **Clear instructions**: Patients must understand their condition, the medicines they need to take, the signs and symptoms to watch out for and when to consult a doctor.

- **Follow-up appointments**: Schedule post-hospital consultations with the gastroenterologist and possibly other specialists.
- **Home care**: If necessary, organise home nursing care, physiotherapy or other health services.
- **Integration with primary care**: Inform the patient's GP of their discharge, their current medical condition and any changes in medication.

3. Patient education and resources
Providing patients with educational resources about their disease, treatments, diets to follow, etc. Education is essential for self-management of the disease.

4. Emotional support
Recognise that discharge from hospital can be a stressful time for patients. Offer resources for emotional support, such as support groups or therapies.

5. Communication
Ensure an open line of communication between the patient and the medical team. This can include emergency numbers in case of complications or concerns.

Discharge planning in gastroenterology involves much more than simply handing over a medical prescription. It requires careful coordination, open communication and ongoing support to ensure patient safety and well-being. By investing time and resources in this process, healthcare professionals can ensure that their patients are well prepared for the next stage of their care.

Patient education for effective self-management.

Patient education plays a key role in gastroenterology. Gastrointestinal conditions, whether common disorders or chronic diseases, can benefit greatly from effective self-management. However, if patients are to play an active role in their own health, they must first and foremost have the necessary knowledge and skills.

1. Understanding the disease
   - **Information about the disease**: Explain the disease in detail to the patient, including its causes, symptoms and likely course.
   - **Visuals and diagrams**: Use images or animations to help illustrate and understand the complex aspects of the disease.

2. Medication management
   - **Precise instructions**: Ensure that the patient fully understands the method of administration, dosage and duration of treatment.
   - **Side-effects**: Information on potential side-effects and what to do if they occur.
   - **Storage of medicines**: Give instructions on how to store medicines, particularly if they require special conditions.

3. Nutritional advice
   - **Specific diets**: Some gastrointestinal disorders may require specific diets. Provide clear guidelines, examples of meals and, if possible, recipes.
   - **Foods to avoid**: Identify foods that may exacerbate symptoms or interfere with medication.

4. Recognising symptoms
- **Symptom diary**: Encourage patients to keep a diary of their symptoms. This can help identify potential triggers and adjust treatment.
- **Warning signs**: Inform the patient of symptoms requiring immediate medical attention.

5. Self-care techniques
- **Relaxation and stress management**: Stress can aggravate many gastrointestinal disorders. Suggest relaxation techniques such as meditation or deep breathing.
- **Adapted exercise**: Suggest adapted physical activities that can help manage symptoms, while taking into account the patient's limitations.

6. Psychological support
Some gastrointestinal conditions, particularly chronic inflammatory diseases, can have a psychological impact. Refer the patient to appropriate resources, such as support groups or therapies.

7. Personalised action plan
Each patient is unique. Work with them to develop an action plan tailored to their needs, symptoms and lifestyle.

Patient education is the cornerstone of self-management in gastroenterology. Not only does it improve patient compliance and quality of life, it also reduces complications and hospitalisations. Nurses play a vital role in this process, as they are often the closest link between doctor and patient. By investing in education, we give patients the tools to become informed players in their own health.

Long-term monitoring and the importance of continuity of care.

The management of gastrointestinal disorders does not stop when a patient is discharged from hospital or at the end of a specific course of treatment. For many patients, gastroenterology requires long-term follow-up to ensure the best possible quality of life and prevent or minimise complications. Continuity of care, which ensures uniform and consistent management, is at the heart of this process.

1. The need for long-term monitoring
   - **Monitoring chronic conditions**: Conditions such as Crohn's disease, ulcerative colitis or cirrhosis of the liver require regular monitoring to detect any complications or relapses.
   - **Adapting treatments**: Patients' needs may change. Regular monitoring allows us to adjust medicines or dosages according to symptoms or the progression of the disease.
   - **Preventing complications**: Certain gastrointestinal conditions can lead to severe complications if left unattended. Regular monitoring allows early intervention.

2. Continuity of care: an essential link
   - **Information transmission**: Ensuring smooth communication between the various healthcare professionals (doctors, nurses, specialists) so that everyone involved has the most up-to-date information on the patient.
   - **Patient-caregiver relationship**: An ongoing relationship with the patient fosters trust, which can improve adherence to treatment and the sharing of information.

- **Care coordination**: Ensuring that the recommendations of different specialists are compatible and coordinated.

3. The importance of continuing education
   - **Evolving knowledge**: Patients need to be kept informed of new advances in treatment and disease management.
   - **Self-management**: Providing patients with the tools they need to monitor their symptoms and know when to seek help.

4. Logistical aspects
   - **Scheduling visits**: Organise regular appointments, adapted to the patient's pathology and needs.
   - **Records management**: Ensuring that medical records are kept up to date to facilitate continuity of care, especially if the patient has to see different specialists.

5. The central role of the nurse

The nurse often plays the role of coordinator in long-term follow-up, being the first person patients contact if they have a problem. Their role is essential for :
   - Regularly assess the patient's situation.
   - Liaising between the patient and the doctor or other specialists.
   - Providing ongoing education and answering patients' questions.

Long-term follow-up and continuity of care are fundamental to ensuring optimal care for gastroenterology patients. By ensuring regular, appropriate and coordinated follow-up, it is possible to significantly improve patients' quality of life and prevent many complications. The nurse, at the heart of this approach, is an essential pillar in ensuring continuity and quality of care.

Chapter 20
CONCLUSION:
THE FUTURE OF NURSING
IN GASTROENTEROLOGY

Technological innovations
and their impact on the business.

Over the years, medicine has seen countless technological advances, each with a significant impact on the way care is delivered. Gastroenterology, as a medical speciality, is no exception. For nurses in this field, these innovations are changing not only the way they provide care, but also the way they interact with patients, the medical team and the technology itself.

1. The advent of capsule endoscopy
   - **Description: This is a** small capsule fitted with a camera which, once ingested, travels through the digestive system and transmits images in real time.
   - Impact on the business :
      - **Less invasive**: Reduces the need for more invasive endoscopies.
      - **Training**: Nurses need to understand how it works and be able to instruct patients in its use.
      -
2. Robotics and surgical assistance
   - **Description**: Surgical robots such as the da Vinci allow more precise and less invasive operations.
   - Impact on the business :
      - **Technical support**: Nurses can be trained to assist with robotic procedures.

- **Accelerated recovery**: Post-operative care can be modified because the procedures are often less traumatic for the body.

3. Telemedicine
- **Description**: Remote consultations via video platforms.
- Impact on the business :
  - **Extended access**: Enables nurses to reach patients in remote or hard-to-reach areas.
  - **Ongoing training**: Nurses need to be trained in tools and software, as well as in effective virtual communication.

4. Artificial intelligence and data analysis
- **Description**: Using AI to analyse data, predict disease and personalise treatment.
- Impact on the business :
  - **Informed decision-making**: Nurses can use algorithms to help identify problems quickly.
  - **Ethics**: Questions around data confidentiality and the interpretation of AI results.

5. Portable applications and devices
- **Description**: Devices that monitor symptoms and eating habits, and monitoring applications for patients.
- Impact on the business :
  - **Real-time monitoring**: Allows nurses to monitor patients' progress and symptoms in real time.
  - **Education**: Nurses must guide patients in the correct use of these technologies.

As technology continues to advance at an unprecedented rate, the role of the gastroenterology nurse is evolving accordingly. These professionals must not only be up to date with the latest innovations, but also be prepared to adapt and evolve with them. Although it may seem daunting, these technological advances promise to improve patient care, making the profession even more rewarding.

Future challenges
and the need for ongoing training.

As medicine advances, so do the challenges facing healthcare professionals. In gastroenterology, nurses find themselves at a crossroads between rapid technological change, new drug treatments, and an ageing global population with increasingly complex healthcare needs. In this context, the need for continuing education becomes all the more crucial.

One of the striking realities of modern medicine is the speed with which information and techniques evolve. Gastrointestinal diseases, for example, are better understood today than they were a decade ago, thanks to advances in genomics and molecular biology. This means that yesterday's treatments may no longer be the most effective or appropriate today.

Nurses must also adapt to the increasing use of technology in gastroenterology. From telemedicine to robot-assisted endoscopy, these tools can improve precision and efficiency, but they also require a new set of skills. Without ongoing training, there is a risk that nurses will find themselves overwhelmed by the tools they are expected to master.

The ethical and regulatory landscape in healthcare is also evolving. Questions about data confidentiality, informed consent in a digital world, or the ethical dilemmas posed by new treatments or technologies, mean that nurses need to be constantly up to date to offer respectful care that complies with regulations.

Continuing education also enables nurses to maintain their certification and membership of professional bodies, ensuring that they meet the highest standards of the profession.

However, beyond the simple need to keep up to date, there is a deeper imperative to continuing education: dedication to excellence in care. Patients expect to be cared for by competent and knowledgeable professionals. By engaging in continuing education, nurses demonstrate not only their commitment to their own professionalism, but also to the health and well-being of their patients.

Ultimately, the future challenges of gastroenterology, whether technological, ethical or medical, underline the importance of continuing education. For nurses, this ensures that they remain at the forefront of their field, offering the best possible care to those who need it most.

Motivation and encouragement for aspirants to this exciting profession.

When considering a career in the medical world, it can be easy to become overwhelmed by the multitude of specialities and roles available. However, for those who are intrigued by the complexity and importance of the digestive system, and want to make a tangible difference to patients' lives, a career as a gastroenterology nurse is an exceptionally rewarding path.

The role of the gastroenterology nurse is both varied and specialised. You will have the opportunity to be involved in diagnosis, therapeutic interventions, treatment management and patient education. This will enable you to acquire versatile skills while specialising in a discipline that is constantly evolving due to medical advances.

It's a field where technology meets humanity. If you are passionate about the latest technological advances, you should know that gastroenterology is at the cutting edge of many medical innovations. But technology aside, human contact remains essential. As a nurse, you will often be the first point of contact for patients, guiding them through their medical journeys, reassuring them in their moments of anxiety and celebrating with them their victories, big or small.

The complexity of gastrointestinal disease also means that every day is different. Every patient brings a new challenge, a new puzzle to solve. This daily dynamism is stimulating and offers unparalleled professional satisfaction, because you know that every action you take contributes to improving someone's quality of life.

What's more, this speciality gives you the opportunity to work closely with a multidisciplinary team of healthcare professionals. Learning is continuous, both from formal training and from exchanges with your colleagues.

And, let's be honest, despite its importance, gastroenterology is often an area that is poorly understood or neglected by the general public. By choosing this path, you are putting yourself at the forefront of raising awareness, educating and, above all, bringing quality care to those who need it.

Finally, remember this: every time you help a patient navigate the complexities of their digestive system, every time you bring comfort, every time you apply your knowledge to solve a problem, you are making a difference. This ability to positively influence the lives of others is a privilege, a responsibility and, without doubt, a source of immense satisfaction.

So, to those of you who aspire to join this speciality, know that the adventure that awaits you is rich, rewarding and profoundly human. Embrace this career with passion and dedication, and you will undoubtedly discover one of the most rewarding paths in the medical world.

www.ingramcontent.com/pod-product-compliance
Lightning Source LLC
Chambersburg PA
CBHW062314290526
45794CB00005B/1807